P9-CSG-618

Pure & Simple
Natural
Weight Control

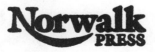

by
Dr. Norman W. Walker
D.Sc., Ph.D.

The Originator Of The

Food Combination
Health Plan

Norwalk
PRESS

Copyright 1981 by Dr. N.W. Walker

All rights reserved. Reproduction in any manner without written permission is prohibited except for brief quotations used in connection with reviews for magazines or newspapers.

Printed in Canada

Published by Norwalk Press
An imprint of Book Publishing Company
PO Box 99
Summertown, TN 38483
(888) 260-8458
www.bookpubco.com

ISBN 10: 0-89019-078-X
ISBN 13: 978-0-89019-078-4

In publishing this book, it is not Dr. Walker's or the Publisher's intent to diagnose or prescribe, but only to inform the reader. Dr. Walker recommends the reader contact a professional doctor specializing in the appropriate subject.

Library of Congresss Cataloging in Publication Data
Walker, Norman Wardhaugh. 1876.
Pure and simple natural weight control.
1. Reducing diets.   2. Food, Natural.
3. Nutrition. I. Title. II. Title: Pure and simple natural weight control.
RM222.2.W263 613.2'5   81-11080
ISBN 0-89019-078-X   AACR2

Book Publishing Co. is a member of Green Press Initiative. We chose to print this title on paper with postconsumer recycled content, processed without chlorine, which saved the following natural resources:

648 pounds of solid waste   13 trees
1,215 pounds of greenhouse gases
5,044 gallons of water   10 million BTU of energy

For more information, visit <www.greenpressinitiative.org>. Savings calculations from the Environmental Defense Paper Calculator, <www.edf.org/papercalculator>.

CONTENTS

Chapter 1
NATURE HAS A WEIGHT-LOSS
PLAN FOR YOUR BODY

Let Nature Be Your Teacher

If you are seeking to have Nature's perfect weight for your body, you must educate yourself to the extent of knowing the full ramifications of putting the wrong kinds of food into your body.

By education, I do not mean the type of information which is often found in weight-loss books or magazines. Some of these "diet" programs can make your life a miserable mess with their complicated instructions and procedures. Throughout the years of my own studies on how the body works, I have found over and over again that Nature's way is best. Man's theories and remedies are complicated; Nature's ways are simple.

If you are carrying excess fat around on your body, you are, indeed, carrying a heavy load which slows down the functioning of the body and depresses the spirit. If you have already been on several weight-loss programs, only to fail after so carefully reading and following the plans, you can only chalk it up to learning by your past mistakes, so that you will not repeat them in the future.

Achieving Nature's plan for your body is simply a matter of concentrating on one line of study, ignoring anything which does not strictly conform to the principles of Nature's laws. If you come to understand and experience eating the foods Nature has provided for your body to work at its maximum efficiency, without carrying that excess load of fat around, you will never again want unnatural and destructive foods to pass your lips.

This education, the elevation of our consciousness of how the body works, is somewhat like that of the person who seeks to eliminate the habit of smoking. If our smoker goes to classes which vividly illuminate the ghastly effects smoking has on the body, he will be shocked into ridding himself of his foul habit forever!

Let Nature Prove Her Plan to You

Throughout this study of how to achieve Nature's perfect weight, I must impress on you the importance of following it through with singleness of mind and purpose. By this, I mean that every word, every sentence and every fact which is related herein must be studied thoroughly without regard to any views or theories which you may have or which others may have set forth. No matter how plausible other presentations of the subject may appear, disregard them completely while you are studying this book.

Remember that there are a great many writers and teachers of weight-loss and health care, many diametrically opposed to the others, yet each claiming to be an authority on the subject. Do not be confused by trying this, that and the other system, until you have proved the truth of the one which will give you the most complete and permanent results.

This Book Is Your Classroom
Your Body Is Your Laboratory

Personally, I have had to learn the truth the hard way (most of us have to do just that!). I am never satisfied with anybody's experiments or recommendations until I have tried them myself and proved it to my own satisfaction.

Everyone wants to have the weight which Nature meant for them, but not everybody wants to do more than wishful thinking or halfhearted attempts at "dieting." I urge you to think of this book as your classroom in which you will grasp the inner meanings of Nature's laws. If you do so, you will find that your body will become your laboratory wherein you will prove that Nature's diet plan will bring perfect and permanent results,

Don't Keep Nature Waiting!

In the following pages I will endeavor to lay out a plan which will allow Nature to mold your body's contour into the shape it was meant to be. I would suggest here, before we begin together to study Nature's ways, that for this program to be effective, you should adopt a positive attitude about its success. There is more truth than fiction in the saying that a person may be down but never out unless he or she chooses. There is really no such thing as a hopeless situation. It is the individual who has grown hopeless about it. I urge you have faith in Nature's ways, for Nature will never let you down.

Chapter 2
FACTS AND MYTHS ABOUT YOUR BODY
How to Diet and Get Fat

Had we been trained from childhood to understand the functions of the body, we would know that the body is composed of billions of microscopic cells.

Microscopic as they are, the cells in our bodies are endowed with life and intelligence. They respond to the stimulus of the mind, whether or not we are conscious of this. They are our servants in every conceivable respect. But in order to carry out their various tasks within our bodies the cells must have food which will nourish them.

In the case of our bodies, Nature has endowed a vast amount of latitude and tolerance in regard to the care that we give to these little servants. When, however, the limit of such tolerance in the manner of nourishment has been reached, we are warned in an indirect manner. We may become tired and fatigued. We may develop headaches and backaches. Even more distressing, we will find that adipose tissue (fat!) has been deposited in those parts of the body where extra fat is neither necessary nor desirable. These "symptoms" are indications that the food eaten in the past was not really of the constructive type, the advertised claims for "diet" foods notwithstanding.

Instead of regenerating the cells of the body, destructive food speeds up the degeneration of the tissues and causes the formation of fat.

An Old Cliche' with a New Twist

There is no question whatever about the fact that we are exactly what we eat. There is no other way in which the cells and tissues of our bodies can be replenished except from the food we eat and the liquids we drink. The irony of this cliche', and it is certainly a true one, lies in the fact that many people in this enlightened age are furnishing their bodies with what they believe to be healthful, nourishing foods. They are eschewing candy, soft drinks and ice cream, eliminating foods with high cholesterol (which their doctors have advised), and cutting down on carbohydrates. What a shame it is to have to tell such people, who are sincerely concerned about their bodies, that they are not providing their bodies' cells with any more nourishment than the person who freely indulges his appetite with all manner of foods.

Does this surprise you? I would be surprised if it does not! The truth of the matter - and I will explain this further on - is that the live cells in our bodies need food that is also alive.

We cannot have death and life at one and the same time. Federal laws prohibit the sale of canned and bottled foods in which life has not been destroyed. When you eat any food which has been preserved or processed by heat, you are eating food in which every vestige of life is missing. This may sound strange to you if you have never stopped to think about it, but as you read the pages of this book, it will become clear to you why the foods you ate in the past did nothing to take unwanted pounds off your figure and certainly did not improve your health.

The fact that for generations millions and millions of people have lived and are living without eating anything but cooked foods does not prove that their being alive is the result of their eating habits. As a matter of fact, they are in a state of decadent existence which is confirmed by the toxic condition of their bodies.

Why else, the overcrowding of hospital facilities?

Why the thousands and thousands of pounds of pain-killers sold annually?

Why such a high rate of heart trouble, diabetes, cancer, emphysema, premature senility and early deaths?

Why are over 15 million citizens of our country overweight?

Why the widespread use of diet pills? (Let me say here to you, never take diet pills. They are dangerous and will cause your body untold harm. Apart from the fact that such medicines are injurious and disrupt the body's metabolism, they do not attack the cause, and at best they are no more than temporary remedies.)

Such conditions arise directly from the state and environment of the cells in our bodies. If we have failed to eat food that would nourish these cells, we have not only starved them, but we have also afflicted them with poisons which the body absorbs from the accumulated debris in the system.

Indeed, yes, we are what we eat. But do we really know what foods we must eat to be what Nature intended us to be?

It is with this in mind that we will now take a look inside our bodies, in order to better understand what kind of nourishment we need to put our food in harmony with our bodies.

There Is a Bomb in Your Body!

As infinitely small as the cells in the body are, each individual cell is composed of atoms and molecules. Millions of these atomic elements are required for the structure of each cell.

Each atom within the cell is virtually a cosmic creation with a terrific volume of power within its core. This was clearly demonstrated in the splitting of the atom in the explosion of atomic bombs such as occurred at Hiroshima on August 6, 1945 and at Nagasaki, Japan, on August 9 of the same year. Even more powerful atom bombs have since been developed, using the hydrogen atom.

The atoms in your system are exactly the same as those which exploded those bombs. Of course, no atoms in your system will ever explode in like manner, although the potential power and energy are nevertheless contained within them!

The number of atoms in your body is beyond your ability to calculate them, yet each atom is virtually a self-contained universe enclosing a terrific amount of energy and power. It is the life-principle in these infinitely microscopic atoms that makes it possible for you to be what you are.

Atoms and molecules are the smallest particles into which matter can be broken down for practical purposes. When two or more atoms are joined together they become a molecule. For example, the chemical formula of water is H_2O, meaning that the smallest particle of water is composed of 2 atoms of hydrogen and 1 atom of oxygen. The formula of the starch molecule is $C_6H_{10}O_6$, meaning that it is composed of 6 atoms of carbon, 10 atoms of hydrogen and 6 atoms of oxygen.

It has been my experience, like that of a great many others, that the body's cells, which are alive with power and energy, must be supplied with food that also possesses that same live, vital energy. Furthermore, this food must be of such a nature that the digestive processes can separate and segregate the atoms and molecules composing it, so that the blood stream and the lymph can carry them to the body's cells for replenishment.

Your Cells are Power-Hungry

If you know anything about growing things in the garden you understand the importance of the care and nourishment which they require to grow and thrive. If they are neglected and do not receive their allotted care, food and water, they wilt, wither and die. Your body is in exactly the same relative situation.

It is vitally important for you to be aware of the kinds of foods which your body needs to nourish it. If the food is constructive, the cells in your body will respond by supplying you with an abundant amount of energy and vitality. You will find that when your cells are properly nourished, you will no longer be attracted to foods that are fat forming and destructive to the body. If you should slip back into eating destructive foods, your body will let you know in a hurry that it does not have the power it needs for maximum efficiency and weight control.

The fundamental purpose of eating is to replenish the chemical elements composing the body's cells. Replenishment is one of the basic laws of nature in regard to organic chemistry. Our physical bodies are laboratories which function under organic chemistry's principles.

Due to the excessive quantity of the inorganic food we eat, we do not properly nourish these cells. Unfortunately, because Nature gave us an elastic body which can take punishment for years on end, man, either through ignorance or indifference, can survive on foods which are appealing to his appetite but are destructive to his body.

The power-hungry cells in our bodies need nourishment which conforms to the Law of Replenishment. This is Nature's basic law for human life. The Law of Replenishment dictates that as each cell furnishes us with its power and energy, it exhausts itself and must be replaced by a new one.

As soon as the atoms and molecules in the cells are worn-out, they are replaced by corresponding atoms obtained from the food we eat. This cycle is constantly carried out within our bodies throughout our lifetime. It is on the quality of this replacement that we build up our health and shed excess fat from our bodies,

Constructive foods, then, are the means by which we keep our bodies functioning to the fullest. Let me stop to say here — and I will say it again and again — that fat people do not know what real health is. How can they? They are feeding their cells with foods that can only produce disorder in the mechanism of their bodies. They must understand that the only way to achieve Nature's perfect weight is to nourish their cells with food that is alive.

How Can We Eat Life?

Life! What does man prize above and beyond everything else? Life! Right?

No scientist, chemist or inventor has ever been able to create life. Life is the sole and exclusive prerogative of our Creator. However, our Creator has given to human beings the privilege of exercising free will.

Self-preservation is the aim of every man, woman and child. Or is it?

Do you know why you eat and drink certain foods? Do you know the difference between food and nourishment?

Do you know what takes place in your system while you are eating, and for hours afterwards?

These and many other questions have a direct bearing on the problem of overweight, sluggish, unhealthy bodies. They are all questions to which we must know the true and fundamental answers. Only then will we be able to intelligently and successfully map out a program of eating and living.

This being the case, is it not intelligent, rational and discerning to conclude that the regeneration and replenishment of the life in your body must essentially come from the life inherent in the food you eat? The life present in such nutrition has the property and the ability to revitalize the life within the cells and tissues of your body.

How, then, can one eat life? Nature's foods, in their natural, raw state contain life within the atoms and molecules that compose them. Such atomic life is classified as enzymes.

Enzymes: As Mysterious as Life Itself
Every plant, vegetable, fruit, nut and seed in its raw natural state is composed of atoms and molecules. Within these atoms and molecules reside the vital elements we know as enzymes. Enzymes are not things or substances! They are the life-principle in the atoms and molecules of every living cell.

The enzymes in the cells of the human body are exactly like those in vegetation, and the atoms in the human body each have a corresponding affinity for like atoms in vegetation. Consequently, when certain atoms are needed to rebuild or replace body cells, there will come into play a magnetic attraction which will draw to such cells in our bodies the exact kind and type of atomic elements from the raw foods we eat.

Accordingly, every cell in the structure of our bodies and every cell in Nature's foods are infused and animated with the silent life known as enzymes.

This magnetic attraction, however, is only available in live molecules! Enzymes are sensitive to all heat above 118°F. At 130°F they are dead. Any food which has been cooked at a temperature higher than 130°F has been subjected to the death sentence of its enzymes, and is nothing but dead food.

Naturally, dead matter cannot do the work of live organisms. Consequently, food which has been subjected to higher temperatures above 130°F has lost its live, nutritional value. While such food can, and does, sustain life in the human system, it does so at the expense of progressively degenerating health, energy and vitality.

This state of affairs is graphically demonstrated when a farmer tries to feed pasteurized milk to a calf. Pasteurized milk is heated at a temperature high enough to supposedly destroy pathogenic bacteria. While the milk is being subjected to high temperatures, all its enzymes are destroyed. As a result, calves fed on pasteurized milk have died within six months!

Fat at Forty: You Don't Have to Let It Happen!

So extremely important is this question of replenishment, that its neglect is plainly visible in the features and on the bodily contours of every man, woman and child. Both indicate that the food eaten in the past failed to furnish the necessary quality of nourishment for the replenishment of the cells. Instead of cell regeneration taking place, cell degeneration has taken place.

In childhood a certain amount of plumpness is tolerated if it is the natural result of a well-balanced diet. But after the adolescent stage has passed, excessive fat and disease are virtually synonymous.

Upon reaching the mature age of the thirties, one's aim should be toward slimness. Such an aim can be achieved by overcoming the habit of overeating and exercising. Exercise and the control of the kind and quantity of food eaten are essential.

If one has reached the forties with a figure that proclaims disinterest in what kind of foods are eaten, that person will join the ranks of 15 million overweight Americans.

It is sad, indeed, to see this pattern over and over again, until the uninformed think nothing of it and regard it as the natural consequences of aging.

With these facts before us, facts which in this enlightened day cannot be contradicted, it is easy to understand why it is so necessary for us to educate ourselves in the ways of Nature.

It is truly difficult, when in a rut, to know just where to turn. Yet our Creator who created us has never yet failed to open the way towards enlightenment. Nature does not establish a law with no means to fulfill it. The resolution of the Law of Replenishment lies within our bodies'cells and in the live enzymes that are found in abundance in Nature's live foods.

Chapter 3
A TESTIMONY FROM A
STUDENT OF NATURE

I Am My Own Guinea Pig!

In my extensive studies in the healing arts during nearly half a century, I have sought to discover the primary cause of human ailments and to find a means to remedy, and more importantly, to prevent them.

Many times my family and friends urged me, to use their own words, to devote my time to something more constructive than to waste it in the type of research into which hospitals and foundations were pouring millions of dollars. Dire effects on my sanity were predicted if I persisted in delving into subjects which were paradoxical to scientific and medical minds.

The Pig Almost Died

When I could see men, women and children all around used as guinea pigs for experiments which to my reasoning and rational mind seemed utterly unnatural, and when I saw these same individuals literally mowed down in a very few years as a direct result of those "accepted scientific treatments" by means of various medical treatments, I was determined more than ever to try to discover the root of our troubles, if it took a lifetime to do it.

From the day I made that decision, I became my own guinea pig No. 1. I decided to live mostly on grain and flour foods, cereals and the like, and I drank large quantities of milk. These foods were generally, and also "authoritatively," proclaimed to be the staff of life complete foods, nourishing foods, foods containing all the essentials for health, strength and what have you.

For two years I was apparently thriving on these foods, when suddenly, one morning I could not get out of bed. I had gained weight, rising from 155lbs, to no less than 197lbs. There was, to all appearances and by accepted standards, nothing whatever wrong with me, until that fateful morning when out of a clear sky I was stricken as if by a bolt of lightning. One doctor after another gave me no hope beyond a few weeks, as cirrhosis of the liver, coupled with the excruciating pains of neuritis, were considered definitely fatal.

Saved by a Friend Who Knew Nature's Ways

I refused to take their medicines or advice. I recalled my talk, a few years back, with a friend with whose wisdom I was deeply impressed. He was a strict vegetarian and told me, "If you should get sick, unable to get up, don't under any circumstances take any drugs. They are poison. Don't eat any food for three days, as sickness is the result of the retention of waste matter in your body. Just drink a glass of pure water every half-hour or so every day, for three days and you will get well."

His remarks struck me forcibly while I lay helpless on my back, and I thought I had nothing to lose and probably much to gain by doing so. He was right.

My friend was as healthy as all outdoors. He ate only raw vegetables and fruits. Why should I not do the same? As I had nothing to lose, I began a regimen of the best raw fruits and vegetables I could find. In six months I was full of energy and ambition, with none of the former ailments that had predicted my demise.

It was this experience which stimulated my research on the relative value of fresh raw foods as opposed to food that is cooked. Again, I became my own guinea pig. When I ate my vegetables raw, I felt well and ambitious, and my bowel movements were quite good. But every time I ate those same vegetables cooked, the next day I slowed down preceptibly. My mind was less alert, and my bowel elimination decidedly less efficient.

An "Egyptian," Playing with Carrots

I again got to wondering. What was there in raw vegetables that caused me to improve so rapidly? I took some carrots and grated them, squeezed the moisture out of them and discovered how much juice there was in them. For nearly a week I did little more than "play" at grating and squeezing the vegetable pulp. Soon I was drinking daily as much as a gallon or more of the fresh, raw carrot juice I was "playing" with.

Doctors had told some of my friends that I could not live more than perhaps a few weeks, yet there I was walking around, as yellow of skin as an Egyptian, yet healthy as could be. Not one of my friends could be induced even to try drinking my juices! It did not take too long for my yellow skin discoloration to disappear, once my liver and gall bladder were in better shape. I learned that the cleansing processes and functions of the liver made me look as if I might have jaundice. It was merely that the large amounts of waste matter accumulated in my liver was dissolving with the help of the carrot juices. Some of the waste matter was being eliminated from my system by way of the pores of the skin.

For a month or so, in my enthusiasm, I was supplying juices to bed-ridden men and women (at my expense) under the supervision of a doctor friend who was tolerant, if not sympathetic, about my theories. The results were excellent, particularly when the patients took to the raw vegetable and fruit diet.

Back to Business As Usual

Of course at that time I was a very young man who knew all the answers. (Did you ever know one who didn't?) I needed money and became engrossed in trying to make a fortune. This soon became my all encompassing obsession and, as is the way of all humans, in the course of two or three years my enthusiastic research and its results not only took a back seat, but in about five or six years that work of regeneration might just as well never have been done. Such is the brevity of the memory of an ambitious young man wallowing in the paths of "big business"

The Same Mistake — Twice

The outcome? Just natural, and what you would expect. A nervous breakdown right at the threshold of the achievement of my ambition. The doctor in London, where my activities were at the time, came to my apartment and told me I had two choices. He told me that if I tried to continue my business activities, my ambitious career would be ended. On the other hand, if I went abroad and abandoned all activities, took a complete rest, in about nine or twelve months I might be able to get back on my feet.

While he was in my room, the doctor saw a woodland picture on my desk. He asked what it was. I told him it was a pen and ink enlargement of a 35 millimeter snapshot I had taken in Brussels about a year earlier. Then I had to confess to him that for the best part of the preceding nine or ten months I frequently enjoyed myself drawing that enlargement, often working until three o'clock in the morning. "Ah," he said, "your trouble is not only business and diet, it is also due to lack of rest and sleep over too prolonged a period of time."

Knowing that I spoke French, he advised me to clear up my affairs in London and, instead of taking a long ship cruise as he had originally suggested, he told me to go to Brittany in the north of France and board with some peasant farmer in order to eat the food they grew and as they prepared it.

Vive La Carotte!

I decided to do as my doctor suggested. I stored my household items and packed my other things for a prolonged stay in France.

When I arrived, I spent a few days looking around Dinan and St. Brieuc, but they were too large for my purpose. My cab driver drove me around, and when we got on the outskirts of the village of Pontivy, I found a charming old couple with a family farm who said they would be glad to accommodate me for about $2.00 a week (in French money of course). They were within comfortable walking distance of the village of Pontivy, a village of 400 or 500 inhabitants — I expect it has grown to be quite a city by now — and not too far from the Aulne River, where I could do some fishing.

This delightful old couple ate mostly raw vegetables and fruits from their garden, which suited me quite well. On Sundays, they killed one of their roosters or a duck. Occasionally, they ate fish from the river.

The Phenomenal Carrot

I was thoroughly enjoying my "dolce far niente" — sweet doing nothing — life, and had noticed some improvement in my strength. One morning, Madame was in her kitchen preparing vegetables and peeling carrots. Watching her, I noticed how moist the carrots were when peeled, even though they had not been in any water. Subconsciously, something flashed into my mind, and later on that afternoon, I asked Madame for permission to pick and peel some carrots. And could I use her grinder? Undoubtedly, she thought this was some queer British idea, but she gladly consented.

Cracking the Code of the Carrot

That afternoon I peeled about a half-dozen good sized carrots. Then I set to work grinding them and straining the pulp through one of Madame's nice clean dish towels. This method was so easy that, forgetful of my previous experience some years earlier, I obtained what I thought was my first introduction to a cupful of excellent carrot juice, made in a matter of seconds.

Each day thereafter, I assumed the job of making juices for myself and for my two hosts, who enjoyed them as much as I did.

The daily drinking of my juice noticeably began to speed up the regeneration of my body. As the days passed I found myself feeling well and strong. The unnatural and unnecessary extra weight I had been carrying around had disappeared, leaving me a figure which reflected my return to health and vitality. As a result, I returned to London in eight weeks, instead of the nine months my doctor had prescribed. Needless to say, he was amazed to see me back and to see how well I looked. He was even more astonished to learn my method of recovery. He considered my eight-week recovery phenomenal.

Nature Gave My Diet Her Stamp of Approval

Since those episodes in my young life, I have advocated a raw vegetable and fruit diet with an abundance of fresh raw vegetable and fruit juices. In addition, my studies throughout the years have shown me without a doubt or question the importance of keeping the body internally bathed by means of enemas and colonic irrigations.

If you are not familiar with these internal methods of cleansing the body of impurities and toxic matter, do not be anxious or mystified. Later on I will give you full and practical instructions. If you should then desire to know more about the colon (the large intestine) and how its condition affects every area of your body, you can pick up a copy of *Colon Health, the Key to a Vibrant Life,* in which I discuss the subject in its entirety.

I can truthfully say that, without exception, every person I have ever known during the past thirty-five or forty years who has gone on such a program has not only been able to overcome weight problems and ailments resulting from the neglect of the body, but has been able to prevent worse calamities, even when surgery was recommended.

The natural reaction many people have on reading this for the first time, is to wonder: If this is true, and so valuable, why does the rest of the world not know it and practice it?

The answer is very simple indeed. The reason it is not generally accepted is due to the impatience on the part of most people who wish to lose weight. They wishfully expect some magic miracle to take place overnight by the use of pills or shots, never considering how long it took to get them into their condition. When the first few attempts fail to show the anticipated or "guaranteed" results, they are apt to flock hither and yon, blindly following other poor souls in similar or worse predicaments, trying whatever remedy happens to have come into fashion.

Impatient to get results without working for them, we are usually not willing to take the necessary time to let Nature work for us doing the job successfully and completely.

Nature takes her time to heal and cure, but the results are lasting. When people appreciate this, understand it, and try it, they learn that Nature wants man to live a life of simplicity. It is man who makes life complicated.

Chapter 4
WHAT DOES NATURE
SAY ABOUT NUTRITION?

1,000 Dead Meals a Year!

Do you really think you can achieve the weight that Nature meant for you? If so, let us seriously consider the problem that confronts you.

In the first place, do you want Nature's perfect weight overnight? It cannot be done, except at the expense of trouble later on. Bear in mind that a home built of brick, stone or wood can be torn down and replaced by another one. Not so with your body. If you neglect your body to the point of no return, you cannot discard it and buy a new one to replace it.

If you are determined to learn the way Nature can take fat off your body, then I have a second question. Do you want to do what is necessary to keep Nature's weight permanently? If so, you will have to work at it systematically according to the plan best suited to your age, to your environment and to the physical health of your body.

To begin with, think how many birthdays you have had since you first saw the light of day. Is it 30, 50, 70, 90?

Next, consider the number of years you have lived and how long it has taken you to get into the condition that you find yourself today. You did not get into this condition suddenly, overnight. No, indeed! You are today the sum total of the food you have eaten all your life, and of the lack of care and attention which you should have given to your body every day of your existence.

You have probably eaten an average of three meals a day, as a matter of habit. That means you have averaged about 1,000 meals a year. If you are forty years old or more, you have consumed more than 40,000 meals in your lifetime, so far.

All Those Expensive Groceries - Gone to Waste!

We will also assume that, like most people, nearly all the food you have eaten as a general rule is the kind everyone else eats. All the food you have eaten has, for the most part, been canned, frozen or likewise processed, and rarely, if ever, have you had a sufficient quantity of raw, fresh food, or a complete meal of nothing but raw vegetables and fruits. Your fare has been what is displayed on the shelves of the grocery store or supermarket, the kind of food that is widely advertised and is thus expensive to buy.

The question, now, for you to ponder, is how many of those meals you ate were actually able to furnish the cells and tissues of your body the real, live vital nourishment they needed for replenishment or regeneration? If you will look at yourself in a full-length mirror, you will find the answer written in every line on your face and neck, in every pore of your skin, and in every contour and outline of your body, and I might add, protruding out in all the wrong places.

It is impossible to regenerate organic (live) cells in the human body with inorganic (or dead) matter. We will find that while the 40,000 meals did serve the purpose of sustaining life, hardly any nourishment in organic form was eaten to regenerate the cells of your body or supply the chemical elements composing them.

Nutrition: The Fuel Your Body Needs to Run On

In understanding what good nutrition really is, we must keep in mind that dead matter cannot do the work of live organisms. The food we eat must not be subjected to temperatures above 130°F. If so, it will have lost its live, nutritional value because its enzymes will be destroyed.

As enzymes form the fundamental basis of nutrition, they should have first consideration in the choice of our food. It bears repeating that enzymes are not substances which man can create, nor are they capable of being synthesized as supplements for use by the body. Enzymes are the life-principle in every live, organic atom and molecule, whether they are in the body or in Nature's vegetation.

In the course of the voluntary and involuntary activities of the body, we expend considerable unconscious energy. This energy is furnished by the enzymes in the atoms of the cells and tissues. When, in this process, the enzymes have carried out their function, the atoms involved are discarded, automatically passing into the blood and lymph streams and are then transferred to the colon for expulsion as waste.

The object, then, of nutrition is to replenish and regenerate the atoms and molecules composing the cells and tissues of the body. Food which is truly nutritious must be replete with enzymes. The enzymes in the body give the spark of activity to every cell and tissue, as well as to their functions, so long as the body is alive. The moment the body dies, the life represented by its enzymes is dissipated, at which time the atoms and molecules and the cells and tissues composing the anatomy are no longer subject to regeneration and begin to decompose.

To sum it up, live replenishment is the sequel to good nutrition.

Man's Ways: Radical/Nature's Ways: Realistic

In order to achieve Nature's perfect weight, many of one's habits must be changed. To do this constructively, one can do it only with an open mind and with the wholehearted desire to see if it really works. I know that Nature will never let you down, but you must prove it to yourself.

A closed mind, working against the tide of mental reservations, a mind which has made it a practice to frown on radical changes in thought, habits and actions is the greatest stumbling block towards any progress on the road to your perfect health, Nature's way.

Unless one can accept, unreservedly, at least on trial, that which most people would consider unorthodox if not actually extreme, it would be almost better to let life take its course, spending the rest of one's days in the familiar ruts of obesity and self-indulgence.

You may be saying as you read this that I am demanding and unreasonable. Let me here assure you that it does indeed take a tremendous amount of courage to decide that you are going to take these steps to rid yourself of excess weight.

It is the coward who sits on a sagging chair in front of a tableful of foods which will not only add more fat to his body, but will ultimately destroy it.

If you are one of the courageous who have searched in vain for a way to lose excess fat, you don't deserve to be victimized by weight-loss claims and statements which are based on half-truths and conventional falsehoods. Moreover, the advertising of weight-loss foods which are constantly put before the public lulls us into believing that the diet foods found on the shelves and freezer sections at the supermarket are healthy and nourishing because they are "low in calories" and claim to have "no sugar added."

Your Body Can Be Reborn — Really!

Once you have discovered the natural means to regain and maintain the weight Nature meant for you to have, you will experience a vitality that may be completely new to you. This increased energy and enthusiasm for life is a promise from Nature if you will heed her ways. Once you have experienced the bliss which results in putting your discovery into daily practice, it will seem to you both strange and pitiful that so many people will not consider the matter. Once you have adopted this way of eating and living you will look at man's ways as radical and at Nature's ways as realistic.

What significance does this have in the diet plans of one who desires Nature's weight-loss program? It is the reassurance that the human body still retains within itself an ability to readjust mental attitudes towards appetites and habits.

Chapter 5
THE BODY, A PERFECT MACHINE, UNTIL...

What Your Body Wishes You Knew About Digestion

In order to understand why Nature prefers certain foods over others, we must make a brief survey of the processes which the foods we eat have to go through, either to be digested and so become nourishment for the cells and tissues of the body, or to become poisons which the body must fight.

Digestion is the essential process by means of which nutrients in the food you eat are assimilated by your body. Naturally, if the food is not properly digested it cannot be completely assimilated and the body is deprived of needed nourishment; at least a part of its nutrition is wasted.

The digestion of food actually begins when the vision or aroma of food alerts the endocrine glands to the fact that the functions and activities of the digestive juices are imminently needed.

As food is anticipated and it catches the eye, the visual and olfactory senses (the eyes and the nose) by the exercise of their role stimulate the endocrine glands into activating the digestive organs, starting with the secretion of the parotid and other salivary glands in the mouth.

Food is better digested when it is agreeably prepared and pleasant to look at. If a food looks unattractive, there may even be a decrease in the secretion of gastric juices.

Mastication and chewing are very important operations, because all solid food must be disintegrated and broken down into a mulch. and our teeth were given to us for that purpose.

Between the mastication by the teeth and mixing of the saliva, the food becomes a bolus (a lump of chewed food) known as chyme, a more or less rounded mass of broken-up food saturated with the saliva, ready for swallowing.

When swallowing, the chyme is propelled through the esophagus into the stomach. The glands in the stomach have, by that time, already been activated to secrete hydrochloric acid for the purpose of disinfecting whatever material is contained in the chyme, thus enabling the chyme to enter into a bath of hydrochloric acid, which begins the process of breaking down the food into simpler chemical materials.

The Pylorus: The Doorkeeper of Your Body

At the exit of the stomach there is a valve which forms a passageway to the small intestine. The pyloric valve controls the volume of semifluids which leaves the stomach after the gastric juices have done their work. It is significant that if only liquids are introduced into the stomach, the pyloric sphincter opens almost immediately and allows the fluid to pass into the small intestine. The pylorus, however, remains closed as long as the food in the stomach is solid. Usually, it takes from three to four and one-half hours before the stomach completely empties a traditional meal of cooked meats, starches, and vegetables into the small intestine! The complete passage of food through the digestive tract takes twenty-four to twenty-eight hours.

Everything that goes down the throat, in the form of food or drink, is broken down into its atomic constituents in the small intestine. The small intestine is equipped with millions of tiny organs like suction cups, called villi, which avidly grab every molecule that can be collected from the material inside the small intestine and pass these molecules to the surrounding blood vessels.

It strains the imagination to try to visualize the millions upon millions of atoms separated from the fiber structure which composed the food, all mixed together in an apparent jumble, streaming through the infinitely small microscopic villi (or tubes) in the walls of the intestine before they can reach the liver.

The Colon: A Frugal Housewife

Once the atomic elements have been liberated from the chyme and are able to pass by osmosis through the walls of the small intestine, it is the blood that transports them, first to the liver through the hepatic vein, then from the liver through the heart for distribution throughout the body, as the liver dictates.

It is at this point that the small intestine passes leftover residue into the large intestine, the colon. The residue is accepted by way of the ileo-cecal valve, which connects the small intestine and the colon. If the colon is clean and is functioning normally, it will take another hour or two for the feces to pass through to the rectum for expulsion.

Although food must pass through some twenty feet of small intestine before its nutritional elements can reach the liver, there is usually still some nourishment in the residue leaving the small intestine to enter the colon. While the function of the colon is to evacuate matter from which the small intestine has extracted nourishment, there nevertheless always remains some particles of nourishment in the residue. Consequently, it is the function of the first half of the colon to extricate from its contents whatever nourishing elements are present in it, transfer them by osmosis into the blood, which, in turn, transports them to the liver.

Do You Know Just How Important Your Glands Are?

There are three endocrine glands that aid in the digestive processes: the liver; the pancreas; and the gall bladder. Altogether there are eight principal endocrine glands involved in the body's functions.

The importance of the endocrine glands is appreciated when you realize they are involved in every function and activity of your body.

If you consider the vast number of ailments in the liver alone - constipation, diarrhea, hemorrhoids, gall stones, jaundice, diabetes, depression, nausea, billousness, abcesses, warts and sclerosis - it makes sense to be informed about these important glands, which, unfortunately, most people are not aware of.

It is a particularly important subject to one who wishes to attain Nature's diet, because the endocrine glands must have compatible conditions of nutrition, of intercommunication one with another, and of cleanliness, otherwise their efficiency is impaired. The energy which enables the endocrine glands to operate comes from the atoms composing them, together with the atoms in the foods we eat.

If you want to learn more about the glands in your body, what they do, and how you can keep them in good working order and free of disease, I would recommend that you get a copy of my book, *Vibrant Health,* as it would be impossible to treat the whole subject here.

In studying *Vibrant Health* and learning about the endocrine glands, you might be surprised to find out that honey is the most constructive nourishment for the liver. The fresh juice combinations for the liver are raw carrots, beets and cucumbers. These are basic liver-food ingredients!

The miraculous operation of digestion is possible because of the regulation and control exerted by the endocrine gland system. Each gland, in its own sphere of activity, exerts its influence on the functions evolving within the liver.

For now, we must take a look at the effect the foods we put into our mouths have on these glands during the process of digestion. Once we understand what happens when we put "conventional" foods into our bodies, we may be amazed that we have never heard this before!

It is always wise to not base your knowledge on habit or tradition. Learn to know the truth before you ever jump to conclusions. No human mind is ever on the same plane after the truth is learned.

Broken-Down Food: Broken-Down Bodies

The liver is one of the most important laboratories in the body. Every particle of food we eat, and everything we drink is broken down into its component parts and carried by the blood to the liver. Here, in its microscopic cells, the atoms and molecules of our food are reconstructed into material which the body uses to replenish, rebuild and repair cells and tissues.

Cooked and processed foods cause the liver to vastly overwork. The atoms and molecules in such foods have become inorganic by virtue of the heat used in cooking and processing. This supply of inorganic, lifeless material is devoid of the magnetism that is needed to attract the atomic elements from the food to the needy cells of the body.

When we eat raw vegetables and fruits and drink fresh juices daily, the activity of the liver is normal. It then carries on its work of cleansing and construction in a thoroughly well-regulated manner. The atoms and molecules in their new form and arrangement are sent on their way into the blood stream for distribution to the glands and to all the other parts of the body. The byproduct of this work is not wasted. Together with the used up cells from the blood and from other parts of the system, the liver converts them all into bile. The bile is collected in the gall bladder for storage where it is used as needed, in many of the activities and functions of our bodies.

Your Liver Has a Mind of Its Own

We will later on be discussing the source of proteins in the diet Nature intends for us, but, for now, let me caution you that it is useless to eat a "complete protein."

What is a complete protein? A complete protein is found in the flesh of animals, fish and fowl and contains all twenty-three of the amino acids.

What are amino acids? Amino acids are chains of atoms which combined act not only as building blocks for the construction of protein, but also have certain active functions which they perform, so long as there is life in the atoms composing such protein.

In other words, amino acids are not only the building blocks making up the protein, but comparing them to an office or any other building, figuratively speaking, they represent all the activities that go on in such buildings.

The Complete Protein Is Not Complete In Our Bodies

It is vital for anyone who is starting on Nature's diet to remember that a complete protein, as such, cannot be digested and assimilated in the human system as a complete protein, whether it is animal flesh or other, irrespective of the number of amino acids composing it.

20

The protein composing the flesh of animals, fish or fowl was obtained from the live, organic atoms in the live vegetation they were nourished with. Such flesh, at this point is a complete protein. When we eat flesh, however, we cannot use either the concentrated protein or the amino acids that compose such flesh. They must all be reduced to the atoms composing them, so that the body may reorganize these atoms to build its own amino acids and proteins.

Nature's Foods Are Always Complete

How much more effective and easier it would have been to avail ourselves of the fresh, raw fruits and vegetables Nature gave us! The very purpose of the creation of the vegetable kingdom was, and is, to give life to atoms. All vegetables and fruits contain the necessary atoms from which amino acids are formed in the human system. The human body cannot utilize for constructive purposes flesh products of any kind in the form of complete proteins, but when we eat raw vegetables and fruits, the digestive organs have virtually no splitting of molecules to do. They merely assist the atoms and molecules to separate, so they can be readily collected by the blood and lymph streams and quickly utilized by the glands, cells and tissues throughout the body.

The liver completely disregards the claims of the manufacturer of "protein products." The liver is not educated to read instructions and promises made by the dispensers of complete proteins.

Do not waste your time or money on complete proteins. Nature's source of protein is less costly and more beneficial.

Your Digestive System Rejects Starches, Hates Sugar and Despises Cooked Fats!

Why Starches?

Only about 7% of all the elements composing your body is in the category of carbohydrates. Classified as chemical substances, carbohydrates are starches and sugars.

There is not one speck of starch in the composition of your whole body, nor can there be, because starch is not soluble in water and therefore cannot be converted into a liquid as a starch. Energy and exertion on the part of the digestive processes are required to convert the starches into natural sugars before the body can use them.

These concentrated starch molecules can cause a colossal amount of damage in the digestive system. When they pass through the liver, the molecules may become wedged in the liver's cells. When this has happened often enough, a congestion results which may readily develop into hardening of the liver (cirrhosis).

When I first realized that the starch molecule was not soluble in water, alcohol or ether, I immediately understood why the grains and starchy foods I had eaten in such quantities in the past caused such impactions in the liver as to cause it to harden like a piece of board. It also gave me a clue as to why gravel and stones sometimes form in the gall bladder and the kidneys, and why the blood coagulates unnaturally in the blood vessels and capillaries, thus forming hemorrhoids, tumors, cancers and other disturbances throughout the system.

Why, then, continue to eat concentrated starches, which are not only unnatural for the body to handle, but also put unnatural, unnecessary weight on your body!

Why Sugar?

To comprehend the danger of using white sugar you must recall that food taken into the mouth takes from three to five hours to travel the twenty feet of small intestine. This sluggish, dawdling pace is necessary for the digestive processes in the intestine to disintegrate every particle of food you eat, and to liquefy it, in order that the atoms composing the foods may pass by osmosis as a liquid through the walls of the intestine and, picked up by the blood, may be transported to the liver.

White sugar does not have the patience to consume all that time to reach the liver. Actually, it becomes a liquid before it has completed its passage through the stomach. Then it fairly pours itself through the duodenum into the small intestine. By the time it has reached only a short way into the small intestine, it has been converted into alcohol and glucose. In this state it flows into the liver, swamping it with an exorbitant volume of glucose. The glucose is then discharged into the blood, causing an excessive amount of sugar to saturate the blood. Sometimes resulting in the blood-sugar affliction known as diabetes.

What Does Fat Have to Do With Globules?

When the glucose content of the liver exceeds its point of tolerance, the liver converts the glucose into fat globules. These fat globules are then discarded from the liver because their retention there serves no useful purpose. What happens to them? Just what you don't want to happen to them! These fat globules are attracted to those muscles in the body which are more or less neglected by a lack of exercise, namely the hips and over the stomach, besides being deposited under the chin.

Usually, on the average, it takes the first thirty years of one's life for these fat globules to change and enlarge the anatomical structure and contour of the victim of the sugar habit, and usually thirty to forty years more before the fat is discarded — in the grave!

Why Cooked Fats?

Basically, fats are combinations of acids, the molecules of which consist of the atomic elements carbon, oxygen and hydrogen. It is the volume and the pattern or arrangement of each of these three elements in the molecules that causes fats to be thin oil, such as vegetable oils, or thick and solid, such as animal fats.

Fats are collected from the intestines by the lymph nodes, but they do not collect any protein or carbohydrate material passing through the intestines. The lymph nodes collect the fats and then convert them into an extremely fine emulsion. In this state they pass it through the lymph channels to the thoracic duct, which is the main lymph channel in the throat, whereupon it is transmitted into the blood stream.

When the fats are cooked, as in fried foods, buttered popcorn and donuts, the fat is converted into an inorganic product, and the process of emulsifying it is far more complicated. This results in the fat remaining in the circulation of the blood, sometimes for hours after eating it, not usable, clogging up the system instead of being available for constructive use.

Any fried flour product, especially one fried in superheated oil, is utterly indigestible. It is virtually impossible for fat-saturated starch to be converted into any of the sugars.

This deleterious combination results in the generation of unhealthy, and needless to say uncomfortable, gas in the system, while giving a curious feeling of fullness and satisfaction at the same time. The end product of the undigested foods cooked in fat is putrefaction and fermentation of the residue by the time it reaches the colon. Malodorus gas, constipation, an offensive bad breath and rolls of fatty tissue in the midriff are the common results of eating such foods as fritters, fried potatoes, griddle cakes and the like. Is the result worth the temporary, and I would say dubious, pleasure of eating fried foods?

Prove Nature's Diet to Yourself

Have you ever noticed how your friends who are in the habit of eating fried foods are looking fatter each passing year, and certainly showing their age much, much sooner than they should? But if they want to eat such foods, it will not do any good to tell them how to become slim and healthy. Of course, that should not prevent you from following the advice you would like to give to them, after having proved to yourself that Nature's diet is perfect!

Fats, though, are a necessary requirement for a balanced maintenance of the functions and activities of the body. Fats form our most valuable reserve supply of energy, just as the storage battery in the automobile has elements in it which enable it to store up the electric current needed to start the engine.

There are many of Nature's foods which give us the necessary fat we need, as I will be discussing later.

Like all other foods, no fats can be utilized by the body until their molecules are broken down into their component atomic elements. When these elements get out of balance, fat will generally be deposited as adipose tissue in those parts of the body where generally they are least desirable.

Knowledge of how the body works and what it needs for replenishment is a step in the right direction. Wisdom, though, is acquired when we put our knowledge into practice.

Do not judge the contents of this book from your own knowledge of what to eat and what to drink. I have given you in these pages the knowledge of Nature's laws. My research has led me to realize that anything to the contrary is the result of man's folly and frailty. The knowledge of Nature's laws, only a fraction of which it is possible to give in these few pages, is imperishable.

Chapter 6
MAN'S ARTIFICIAL FOODS
SUGAR

Man's Fake Food ...

Before I present the first steps you must take for your initial weight-loss, and then, secondly, lay out a plan for eating Nature's food for the rest of your life, we must examine together Nature's foods in relation to man's foods. Do not be discouraged! For every man-made, unnatural food you eat, Nature could have provided a genuine article. With Nature's foods you will never have to worry about your weight, for Nature will tend to your body, keeping it slim and healthy.

Many people, interested in the health of their bodies and the shape of their figures, are beginning to educate themselves as to the harmful effects of sugar. Diabetes has made such a devastating inroad into the health of children, no less than of adults, and the warnings are on the increase. Despite this, many people have a false impression about the efficacy of the different types of sugars available.

Where Does Sugar Come From?

Chemically, sugars are divided into the following classifications, namely: cane, beet and corn. These are man-made, manufactured products, meaning they are processed by intense heat and, being devoid of enzymes, are consequently a food hazard.

Sugar, Sugar, Everywhere, but Don't Eat a Drop!

Later on in this dissertation on sugars I will acquaint you with the contents of additional man-made sugars, which you will find in abundance on the lists of contents on the labels of most canned goods, soft drinks, cheeses, meats, soups, bacon, crackers, bread, cereals and condiments. More importantly, these sugars are used in the composition of "diet foods."

It is necessary for you to understand the classifications of sugars and their purposes, because harmless "natural sugars" are present in the composition of all vegetation. Furthermore, the sweetening of food has become a necessity in order to make certain foods and their combinations more palatable.

The Pure White Drug Crystals in Your Sugar Bowl
Were Once Sugar Canes Growing in Nature's Fields

When man makes sugar from sugar cane, the stalks are crushed and pressed to remove the sweet juices inside them. These raw juices are then processed several times, to reduce them to the "pure" white crystals that eventually reach the dining room table.

During the first process of refinement, when the juice is filtered and treated with chemicals to "remove impurities," molasses remains after the crude sugar has been removed. The molasses then goes through several more "refining" processes, gradually becoming lighter in color. The first stage is a dark brown, moist sugar. But it becomes both lighter and drier in each stage, until it becomes fine-grained, pure white crystals.

Do you know how the chemical heroin is made? Man takes the juice of the poppy and puts it through a refining process. The juice is first refined into opium, then further refined into morphine, and, finally, into heroin.

What heinous crimes man commits against himself, and against Nature!

Sugar: Opening Pandora's Box

The digestion of commercial, industrial white sugar has a damaging, deleterious effect on the teeth, the gastrointestinal tract and the alimentary canal. It also causes intestinal disorders such as diabetes, cancer, affliction of one's vision, pyorrhea, destruction of the tissues of the gums and loss of teeth.

White sugar has a very destructive effect on women, increasing and intensifying pain during menstruation, aggravating nervousness and weakness. While this is generally considered "natural," it is, in fact, utterly unnatural and unnecessary. Complete abstinence from white sugar, substituting honey in its place, has frequently prevented or stopped these discomforts.

Sugar is not only harmful in itself, but when used with fruits of every kind, it destroys their value. Fruits are the cleansers of the body, and even those which are acid to the taste have an alkaline reaction in the system, provided, of course, they are ripe. When sugar is added, however, the chemical action of their digestion is entirely changed and they generate excessive acids in the body.

Did You Know That the Sugar You Swallow
Turns Into Acids and Alcohol?

When we eat sugar in any shape or form, in food, in candy or in liquids, it ferments in the system causing the formation of acetic acid, carbonic acid and alcohol.

Acetic acid is a powerfully destructive acid, as witness its use to burn warts off the skin. If it burns so destructively on the surface of the skin, I shall leave you to figure out the damage it does to the delicate membranes in the intestinal tract. As a matter of fact its effect is very pronounced as it rapidly penetrates the system. Because of its affinity for the fats in the nerve texture, it reacts on the nerves with paralyzing consequences.

The alcohol from sugar is equally destructive, and even more devastating, as it acts as a solvent for elements in the body which are only soluble in alcohol and are difficult to rebuild. It tends to gradually destroy the texture of the kidneys. It also affects the nerves which are closely related to the brain and has the tendency to disrupt the functions of observation, concentration and locomotion, in exactly the same manner that alcoholic beverages do, but of course more slowly.

When Pandora Lifted the Lid, Out Flew
Plagues and Sorrows for Mankind!

When we eat sugar, or drink liquids containing it, as in soft drinks, for example, the effect on the pancreas is exceedingly harmful. The pancreas, nestled in the duodenum (or second stomach), is the most active of our digestive glands.

Through a duct, the pancreas injects into the duodenum the necessary digestive juices which enables us to digest several kinds of food at the same time.

When sugar is introduced into the pancreas it is both overworked and subject to disturbing reactions. Because sugar is a "dead" processed product, the resultant pancreatic disturbances cause many ailments and afflictions.

In the liver, sugar is stored in the form of glycogen. If sugar is constantly introduced into the liver, and it is filled to its maximum capacity, the excess glycogen is returned to the blood stream in the form of fatty acids. Of course, those fatty acids are then deposited in all the wrong places on our bodies.

Sugar Addiction: A World-Wide Phenomenon

While it can accurately be said that sugar is a drug, actually it is a man-made chemical. People who use much of it (and the vast majority can hardly avoid it) go through the same degeneration, sooner or later, that a drug addict goes through.

When Pandora Clapped Down the Lid,
One Good Thing Was Left: Hope.

If you are convinced of the terrible scourge left in the body by eating man-made sugars, and you decide to eliminate sugar in any form in your diet, it is especially important to realize that, because sugar is a drug, you must be careful about going off it in a sudden fashion.

Your body will crave sugar for several days, perhaps even a week, but if you will drink a small glass of orange juice when the sugar "urge" hits you, the craving will be satisfied. In fact, once you have gone without sugar for several weeks, you will look on it with distaste, wondering why you ever ate such sickening sweet foods!

When speaking of the destructive effects of sugar, I refer to the manufactured product. In this category we class the white, brown, raw and every other kind of sugar, including molasses and maple sugar. They all have been processed with heat. The white sugar, however, is the most destructive and degenerating of all, because it is usually "refined" with the use of sulphuric acid.

Apart from all other facts and considerations, the body needs sugar, but it does not need the refined cane, corn or beet sugars. The body needs and constructively uses the sugar Nature provides which is present in raw vegetables, fruits and, best of all, honey.

Honey: A Gift From Nature

When we have need for sweetening, we use honey which has been extracted from the honeycomb, without excessive heat. Honey is a pre-digested sweet, or carbohydrate, which can be used with any fruit or other food.

When we feel an urge for something sweet, we eat dates, figs, raisins and other fruits rich in natural sugar. Nature's sugars will never make us fat!

Be Careful that Your Honey
Has Not Had a Traumatic Experience!

It is an incredible fact, but did you know that if the label on your honey container says, "uncooked," it really has been heated? That is the legal term allowed processors who heat their honey up to 160°F for thirty minutes to kill the yeasts, retard granulation and, in general, make it possible and easier for themselves to bottle the honey! That lovely, crystal clear honey has been heated and processed, deprived of its most essential vital elements, including the pollen. It can be assumed that such heated honey has probably suffered some traumatic experiences since the bees last saw it. The vitamins, minerals and enzymes in live, unheated honey is what we want!

By carefully considering this material I have given you to ponder over, you will appreciate exactly why we completely avoid all manufactured sugars, all foods and liquids containing them, and all candies and sweets.

Nature's Diet Helps You Say, "No!" to a Candy Bar.

When a candy bar containing sugar, for example, is offered to us, we refuse it firmly, as we know that by eating it, we would only be injuring ourselves.

Furthermore, if we ate it, eventually it would prove to us that the appeasing of a sweet tooth is certainly not the way to give Nature all our cooperation in keeping our bodies healthy and slender.

We often hear of trainers giving athletes sugar just before an athletic event. The purpose is to give the individual a shot of extra energy. Both the trainer and the athlete, in such cases, do not realize what happens after the "energy" effect of the sugar is dissipated. As a rule, the athlete is completely exhausted and often even collapses at the end of the event. His body was whipped into activity by the false stimulant, which acted as an explosive. It was just like putting gasoline in an oil stove, because the gasoline contained more heat units, or calories. The result was a destructive explosion.

I was visiting some friends in the East some years ago, whose home was on the banks of a river where college students practiced their sculling, or rowing. I became acquainted with one of the trainers and suggested that at the races he give each of his team a tablespoon of honey just before the start of a race. He did just that. The race was a close one, but while the other team happened to win by a narrow margin, every member on the opposing team collapsed at the end of the race, while every one of the team members who took the honey were able to row back to the clubhouse! The trainer on the opposing team had given each member of his crew three lumps of white sugar just before the race!

Who Needs Sugar? The Food-Processing Industry

And now here is the rest of my list of man-made sugars. Becoming aware of the contents in these sugars should shock you enough to never want these foods or beverages in your house again.

Corn Syrup: A transparent thick glucose which is obtained from corn starch by heating the starch with acids to prevent crystallizing. It is used as a cheap sweetening agent. Corn syrup quickly turns into alcohol in the digestive system and may have the tendency to dissolve fat-soluble vitamins in the body. It also has a predisposition to interfere with the functions of the pancreas, particularly if there is a susceptibility to diabetes.

Dextrose: This is a natural sugar present in animal and plant tissues, but dextrin is man-made commercially by the decomposition of starch by the action of acids. Mixed with iodine, it yields a red color. It is used in the manufacture of adhesives, for sizing, as a substitute for gums, in making soft drinks and in beer. Obviously, such a product can readily cause many types of ailments. Physical and mental disturbances can ensue, as the end product in digestion reaches the area of the brain, interfering with the normal functions of the nerves and muscles, and with the cerebrospinal fluid.

Glucose: In Nature, glucose occurs in the digestion of carbohydrates, but commercially it is made by heating starch — especially corn starch — with acid, in order to make a cheap corn syrup to use in soft drinks.

Saccharin: This is manufactured on a large scale. It is made from coal tar and formed by dehydrating saccharinic acid. While it is from 300 to 500 times sweeter than cane sugar, it has no food value whatever. On the contrary, like every coal tar product, it has a definite acid reaction in the body.

Corn Starch: This is the product of milling corn with a final washing in caustic soda. In the process, the hull and the germ (the germ is a living substance, the embryo of the life of the seeds in plants) are removed. Then they are steeped in a solution of sulphuric dioxide gas to prevent fermentation.

The oil is then extracted and the residue of the germ is made into cakes for fattening cattle and sheep. The starch granules, in their coarse state, are used as cattle feed, while the rest of the granules that form a white flour are cleaned with caustic soda and sold for human consumption!

So, the corn starch, so smooth, fluffy and white, carries with it the effluvium and emanations of caustic soda. As you probably know, caustic soda is commonly used in bleaching, making soap and refining industrial oils. The digestion of corn starch has no constructive purpose. Whether it is used as a starch or in beverages, it tends to clog up the fine filtering tissues of the connective veins and arteries.

Nature Can Satisfy Your Sweet Tooth

Unquestionably, sugar is very important in the function of metabolism. There is always sugar present in the blood stream, which is known as blood sugar, and this is an essential component of the human system. White sugar, however, is no more like blood sugar than a horse chestnut is like a chestnut horse. This applies also to the comparison of white and brown sugar with honey and with the sugar in fresh fruits.

Never be deceived by the expression used in sugar advertisements as pure cane sugar. This expression, pure sugar, in this case means that everything of nutritional value has been removed from the product, leaving a lifeless, useless substance which, when ingested, rushes through the stomach to become alcohol even before the liver has a chance to work on it.

As you begin to experiment with the fresh vegetable and fruit juices (which are listed in their various combinations in the recipe section), will find that there are many that will satisfy a "sweet tooth."

Chapter 7
MAN'S ARTIFICIAL FOODS
STARCH

Fast Food is Fake Food

In this day and age, starch has become a commonplace item in most of the foods we eat. We have become so familiar with its abundant availability, that we are no longer conscious of the large amounts of it that we eat.

As this is the age of "fast food," the ease with which we can get a quick meal is taken so much for granted that we rarely stop to think about the ingredients in it. The fact that young people are consuming vast amounts of sweet and sugary starch products is either an indication of our apathy or our lack of knowledge.

Did you ever observe people selecting their purchases of groceries? They go from isle to isle, picking up a little of this and a handful of that, without reflection or observation, stuffing food items into an overloaded grocery cart and off they go. They have not the vaguest idea of the ingredients in the food they are buying. Their carts are packed with boxes and sacks of starch, much of which is hidden in the list of ingredients on food items. If they would begin to read the labels on the bottles, cans and packages they buy, it just might shock them into taking some positive steps towards learning about the superiority of Nature's foods.

A Concentrated Starch Will Make You Fat
A Natural One Will Never Add a Pound

It is of the greatest importance, if we are wanting to put only natural starches into our bodies, to learn the difference between a concentrated starch and a natural one. Then we can always be sure we are eating Nature's perfect foods, not man's substitutes.

Man's substitute starches are dehydrated in the sense that the water content has been dissipated. These concentrated starches have been treated to remove what mankind has decided is "inessential." Thus all processed products made with flour, such as bread, cakes, crackers, spaghetti and other pasta are classified as concentrated starches. They are not only devoid of any water content, but in their preparation they have been either cooked, fried or heated, thus destroying the enzymes Nature intended for the regeneration of your body's cells.

Do You Know You May Be Eating Dehydrated Paste?

It is impossible for man to improve on Nature by removing vital elements from foods and replacing them with manufactured products. If you are not familiar with the process by which man-made starch products are manufactured, please take an unbiased look at how macaroni, or pasta is made. Also keep in mind that what seems like a perfectly normal food, one that everyone eats, does not make it a food which Nature has planned on you eating.

In the manufacture of macaroni and other pasta, the wheat is first ground into a meal, and the bran (the outer coating of the grain of wheat, which is rich in vitamins and minerals) is removed. The second principle ingredient is water, which is added to the flour, and kneaded into a dough. (These two ingredients, flour and water, have for generations been used by mothers to make "homemade" paste for their young children to use in art projects, such as making scrapbooks and the like!)

Pasta Production: Children's Games With Dough

If the pasta is going to be the long, thin kind, the dough is forced through a mold into a tube shape. Other varieties are made by stamping dough into shell-shapes, little stars, circles, hollow tubes and "ribbons." The shaped dough is then dried in special rooms where the temperature is controlled to speed drying. What do we have by the time this product reaches the shelves of the grocery store? A package of dehydrated, concentrated starch.

Man-Made Starches Have Their Uses, But...

Starch is used by mankind in an infinite variety of ways. It is used as a binder and strengthener in making cloth. It is used to thicken colors and also in mixing substances to make paper, medicines, toilet powders and in china clay. It can be said that starches are all very fine and useful, but — why are we eating them?

Our bodies try to tell us that this man-made, artificial food is abnormal, but we are too occupied with our ailments and our overweight bodies to realize that these problems are Nature's warnings that man-made foods are deleterious to our health and our figures.

Nature Doesn't Play "Let's Pretend."

How does Nature provide us with starches? When carbohydrates (sugars and starches) are nourishing and compatible, they can only come from Nature's goodness. In Nature, both sugars and starches are formed in green plants. The carbohydrates which Nature considers nourishing are vegetables and fruits, potatoes, beans, lentils, herbs,

33

peas, grains - when eaten raw. Beans, peas, lentils and grains, when sprouted, are superior carbohydrates.

If you are concerned about the preparation of these foods in their raw states, please do not be alarmed or dismayed. Fixing these foods and their juices are very simple, and you will find yourself enjoying them after you have tried some of the varieties of salads and the vegetable and fruit juice drinks in the back of this book. You will find that your taste for man-made sweets and starches, those foods that will make you fat, will be satisfied by eating Nature's foods instead.

As you are adjusting to this new way of thinking and eating, remember that many of one's habits have to be changed. To do this constructively, one can do it only with an open mind and with a wholehearted desire to see if it really works.

A closed mind, working against the tide of mental reservations, a mind which has made it a practice to frown on radical changes in thought, habits and actions is the greatest stumbling block toward any progress Nature has to give.

You Can Cooperate With Nature by Unlearning
What You Have Always Believed

It is an easy matter to remember the differences between natural and concentrated foods if we have perceived through this study that Nature's vegetables and fruits contain sugars and starches as well as proteins! And that Nature will provide a 100% superior product!

Does this surprise you? If it does, you are in the company of a great many people who think that the only way they can get protein is from animal flesh, especially if they have tried all-protein, weight-loss diets. Most dieters fail to avoid sweets after the second day of "dieting," as they are feeling the withdrawal symptoms from the lack of sugar. Starches are so much a part of our eating habits, eating habits, that it is impossible to avoid them when on a "conventional" diet.

Wouldn't it be easier if these "dieters" knew that Nature could provide them with a source of sugars, starches and proteins that contain the finest nourishment in the world, and, in addition, eating these foods would allow Nature to automatically monitor their weight.

At this point, it would be a good idea for you to turn to the back of this book to the section titled, *Vegetable Value Chart.* As you look through these pages, you will find the compounds (carbohydrates, sugars and starches), and the vitamins and minerals that are found in all fruits and vegetables. As you begin your natural food diet, it will be of help in reassuring you that you are getting all the food elements you need.

It is imperative for us to know the difference between natural and concentrated foods. If we are aware of where each food comes from and how the body processes them, we will be highly motivated to never again put any manmade, concentrated foods into our mouths!

Where Have All the Real Foods Gone?

When you seriously undertake the steps necessary to regenerate your physical body, you become aware of the ease with which one slips into the negative line of least resistance in the matter of nutrition, with no concern as to the kind and quality of the food one eats. One day, you begin to look around, and suddenly you wonder how people (maybe yourself, also!) have managed to live as long as they do on the destructive diets and other undeniably noxious foods and beverages used to appease the appetite. You wonder how people can exist on the artificial foods man has concocted for himself.

White Flour — The Staff of Death

Did you ever stop to think about the bread you eat? Most of you are probably not aware of the evolution of white bread, and, because it is vital for you to know why you should never eat it, I will hope to make you aware of its great danger.

Grains contain the largest concentration of starches, and that is where the problem lies. Up to 140 years ago, there was no such thing as the "white flour" of today. All flour coming from the flour mills was plain "whole flour," with all its inherent natural, nutritional elements retained.

Hungary, the foremost flour producing country in Europe at that time, began using machines equipped with rollers to crush the grain, breaking down the cell structure. Further development resulted in the production of fine, white flour, followed by the Viennese bakers specializing in what became known then, and is still known today, as Vienna rolls.

As usual, Americans were quick to capitalize on the European fad for Vienna rolls. The year 1880, or thereabouts, saw the Minnesota wheat industry embark on the production of white flour which, year after year, became more and more devitalized.

What a paradox that for 4,000 years people used whole grain exclusively, and when civilization entered into a so-called period of progress, nearly every vestige of life was taken out of the bread they ate daily!

Sylvester Graham — A Man Ahead of His Time

One of the foremost exposers of the danger which civilization faced in the use of devitalized white flour was Sylvester Graham, the great temperance and pure food advocate, born in 1794 and died in 1851. He advocated the use of the whole grain, unbolted and coarsely ground in the making of bread and other baked products. His specialty, Graham Bread, is still being produced and used to this day.

At that time it was amazing to read syndicated stories by doctors proclaiming the virtues of "refined" white flour products, declaring them to be nutritious in the face of all contrary proof! On the other hand, there were many prominent physicians who denounced the practice of devitalizing flour as a step toward the deterioration of peoples' health. How farsighted they were, and how true this has turned out to be!

A Refined, Elegant Corpse

Today, bread and all starchy foods sold in the supermarkets are made mostly from "refined" flour. To many people the word "refinement," means elegance, loveliness, grace, neatness, clean and similar qualifications. To those who are conscious of nutrition, the word "refinement" when used to describe white flour, means the food has been robbed of everything of constructive value,

To salve their consciences, the millers and manufacturers have added useless products and chemicals to "fortify" the flour and its products. "Refined" white flour is dead. I have never yet heard of a corpse being fortified to convert it into anything but a corpse.

Toast: Throw It, But Don't Eat It!

At one of my lectures, an amusing, little old lady heard me hold forth against starches, especially bread. During the question period, she stood up and proudly said, 'I toast my bread in my oven until it is thoroughly dry and hard. Don't you think that is much better?"

"My dear lady," I could not resist answering, "neither one is good for you. However, if you make toast out of your bread, when you throw it out your window, it will go much farther than the untoasted one."

The Foundation of Knowledge Is Laid By Study
Wisdom Comes From Its Application

Since so many people are still accustomed to eating white bread and other white flour products (although there is an encouraging resurgence in our country for whole grain foods), I will take a little time here to explain why you should take a closer look at that soft, white, completely devoid of nutrient value, bread.

The outer coatings of the grains which should not be removed are composed of some of the most essential vitamins needed for the maintenance of health. To name a few, biotin, riboflavin and nicotinic acid, without which malnutrition and other ailments result.

There are a few ailments which have been definitely proven to result from eating excessive amounts of devitalized flour products: dilation of the heart; acute anemia; swollen legs and paralysis.

Words are inadequate in expressing the grave danger of the consumption of baked foods made from devitalized white flour. Such foods have no place whatever in the diet of one who aims to be slim and healthy, Nature's way.

How You Can Have Your Grain and Eat It Too!

For one who simply cannot give up grains, there is a method you may use to prepare them, especially if you enjoy grains in the morning for breakfast. (In the recipe section you will find other suggestions for breakfasts.)

Whole grains need not be cooked. They can be soaked in hot water (120°F) overnight. (We use a wide-mouth Thermos bottle.) Be sure in your preparation that you never bring the water to a boil. When sufficiently soft enough to be chewed comfortably, they can be eaten with a little honey as a sweetener. They should never be sweetened with sugar! Eating some sprouted seeds with them is truly good and beneficial.

Eat just a small amount at a time. Remember that the first process of starch digestion begins in the mouth. Hold the grains in your mouth until they are thoroughly saturated with saliva, then chew them up until they are liquified before swallowing. Just take your time. If you have never tried this, I think it will be a revelation to you.

After becoming accustomed to this food for a few days, I expect you will be looking forward to this delicious item with which to start or to supplement your daily breakfast.

The grains we would recommend using are oats, rye and wheat, trying whenever possible to purchase organically grown unprocessed seeds, avoiding the commercial, agricultural, "treated" ones. Such treatment is designed to prevent and destroy diseased plant organisms.

As far as obtaining organically grown foods, it would be a mistake to be fanatical and overly fussy about the quality of the foods we are obliged to purchase at the markets. When we are able to obtain organically grown food, we feel fortunate but, generally speaking, if you are not able to buy exactly the food you want, then as long as it is necessary to do so, take the best of what is available.

Just be sure that you pick the freshest and best quality you see. In addition to grains, this, of course, applies to whether you are buying vegetables and fruits for salads, or for making juices.

A study of the contents of this book will, I am sure, if put into practice, convince the most skeptic that, while the human system needs minerals in its nourishment, emphasis should center first and foremost on the selection of nourishment in relation to the needs of the body. The needs to satisfy the appetite is a different matter. Appetite is the craving of the mind, whereas hunger is the call of the cells of the body for nourishment.

Don't Let Your Appetite Bell Ring

If you want, you can satisfy your appetite with whatever your craving dictates. In that case the kind and nature of the foods you eat and drink is of little consequence, if you don't care. When satisfaction is the result of eating and drinking what is incompatible for the welfare of your body, you cannot blame anyone other than yourself for the consequences. In that case you are the victim of your uncontrollable cravings.

When you have learned to control your appetites and your cravings, and center your choice of food on what will regenerate and replenish your system, you will be giving the cells and tissues of your body the live enzymes they need. They, in turn, will bless you with health, energy, vigor, vitality and a longer life.

Obesity is rarely the result of hunger, but it is definitely associated with the mind responding to the desires of appetite. Thus we understand why appetite can be under the control of the will power.

In my experience over many decades, as well as in the experience of a great many other investigators and researchers, breads, cakes, cereals and other cooked, starchy foods can be blamed for a vast majority of the ailments that afflict today's civilization. I cannot emphasize too strongly that the best proof anyone could want would be to try eliminating such foods from the diet for two to three weeks to give the body a chance to rehabilitate itself. You will be delighted to see your bodyweight decreasing and your health and vigor increasing!

Chapter 8
MAN'S ARTIFICIAL FOODS
FATS

Even If You're Fat, You Need Fats

Fats are a necessary requirement for a balanced maintenance of the functions of the body. Chemically, fats are a combination of glycerin and one or more fatty acids. Fatty acids are composed of the atomic elements carbon, hydrogen and oxygen.

But You Need to Eat Only Nature's Fats!

Fats are divided into three classes:

1. Thin oils such as vegetable oils, namely sunflower seed oil, sesame seed oil, rice bran oil, safflower oil, walnut oil and olive oil.
2. Thick, heavy oils such as animal fats.
3. Grease, such as Crisco, lard and other shortenings.

A Grease-Filled Onion Ring —
What Has Man Come To?

Humanity is hurtling headlong towards disaster as they consume untold millions of deep-fat fried doughnuts, french fries, ghastly fried onion rings covered with dough, fish, also with a coating of dough and bread crumbs. They are absorbing huge quantities of grease into their bodies with the consumption of fried hamburgers, pancakes, eggs, potato cakes, bacon and a whole list of many other items, which I have neither the space nor the inclination to go into.

Your Body Needs Lubrication, Just Like Your Car

One of the functions of fat is to lubricate the joints in the bone structure of the body. With the phenomenal increase in the consumption of foods cooked in hot oil and grease, there has been a corresponding and alarming rise in the number of people having trouble with pain in their joints, caused by the drying up of the lubricant known as sinovial fluid, which is secreted into the joints to keep them supple and free.

Make Sure You Know How To Keep Your Fat
In Your Liver and Not on Your Hips

The laws of chemistry apply to our food no less than to our digestive process. In order for the fats we eat to be digested they must be split up into glycerin and into the atomic elements of the fatty acids. Emulsification (the splitting up of the fatty acids) takes place as the bile and the pancreatic digestive juices supply the necessary atomic elements of sodium and other free alkaline atomic elements.

After being emulsified, the product is transferred to the liver for absorption and reconversion into natural fats. Thus, the liver both stores and distributes natural fats. However, if the fats have been heated in excess of 125°F, they will fail to be adequately treated by the pancreatic digestive juices and will not be available for use by the liver. They are wasted.

Lard, margarine and similar packing house products, fats, oils and greases, have been subjected to very high temperatures in order to process them. Thus, their constructive nutritional value is totally destroyed.

The temperature of oils and fats used for cooking food varies from 350°F to 450°F. Olive oil, for instance, when used to fry food, is readily heated to about 350°F, at which temperature it decomposes. It is the same with similar oils.

The fuel which the body runs on is the result of the food we eat combining with oxygen to produce combustion. The heat resulting from this combustion produces energy.

The atomic elements iron and sodium are among the elements necessary to enable the blood to use sufficient oxygen for the complete combustion of the carbon in the fatty acids. Failure to accomplish such combustion results in the accumulation of excessive amounts of fatty tissues, where they are least desirable. Such a condition also affects the digestion and assimilation of proteins and carbohydrates, which are then also diverted into the formation of adipose tissue.

You will find the following list of atomic chemical elements and their sources to be helpful in eating those foods which are consistent with the chemical needs of your body.

Atomic Elements and Their Sources

Oxygen: Breathe deeply to obtain free oxygen and drink as much fresh, raw juices of fruit and vegetables as possible to obtain organic oxygen.

Carbon: Nuts, especially unsalted almonds, but not peanuts (peanuts are exceedingly acid-forming). Nut butters are very good if raw but not when heated in any manner whatever. Olives and avocados are excellent sources of carbon. Butter (unsalted) and cream are also good sources, when not pasteurized.

Hydrogen: Carrots, celery, spinach, cabbage, lettuce, tomatoes, grapes, huckleberries, red raspberries.

Nitrogen: Breathe deeply and rhythmically in open spaces. Alfalfa and other green leafy vegetables are also sources.

Calcium: Almonds (unsalted), carrots, dandelions, turnips, spinach, oranges, goat's milk (raw) for infants, okra, cauliflower, tomatoes, garlic, parsnips, all berries, all nuts (except peanuts), apples, potatoes (raw), apricots.

Phosphorus: Kale, parsley, radishes (large white), asparagus, sorrel, watercress, Brussels sprouts, garlic, Savoy cabbage, carrots, cauliflower, squash, cucumbers, leeks, lettuce, turnips, Brazil nuts, walnuts, huckleberries, blackberries, cherries, black Mission figs, oranges, limes.

Potassium: Carrots, celery, parsley, spinach, beets, cauliflower, leeks, garlic, raw potatoes, sorrel, squash, tomatoes, turnips, oranges, lemons, apricots, bananas, cherries, dates, grapes, huckleberries, figs, pears, peaches, plums, raspberries, watermelon, pomegranate, olives.

Sulfur: Brussels sprouts, watercress, kale, horseradish, cauliflower, cabbage, chives, garlic, sorrel, cranberries, raspberries, pineapple, currants, apples, Brazil nuts, filberts.

Sodium: Celery, carrots, spinach, tomatoes, strawberries, radishes, squash, lettuce, dandelion, leeks, cucumbers, beets, turnips, apples, apricots, watermelon, huckleberries, pears, oranges, grapefruit, lemons, dates, cherries, grapes.

Chlorine: Beets, cabbage, celery, garlic, horseradish, parsnips, sweet potatoes, tomatoes, avocados, dates, pomegranate, coconut.

Fluorine: Almonds (unsalted), carrots, beet tops, turnip tops, dandelion, spinach, celery tops, goat's milk (raw), Swiss cheese, egg yolks (beat up raw with honey in orange juice), cauliflower, cabbage, watercress, parsley, cucumber.

Magnesium: Carrots, celery, cucumbers, almonds (unsalted), dandelions, garlic, leeks, kale, lettuce, tomatoes, spinach, lemons, oranges, apples, blackberries, bananas, figs, pineapple, Brazil nuts, pecans, pinons, walnuts.

Iron: Lettuce, leeks, carrots, dandelions, radishes, asparagus, turnips, cucumbers, horseradish, tomatoes, almonds (unsalted), avocado, strawberries, raisins, figs, watermelon, apricots, cherries, huckleberries, walnuts, Brazil nuts, apples, grapes (Concord particularly), pineapple, oranges.

Manganese: Parsley, carrots, celery, beets, cucumbers, chives, watercress, almonds (unsalted), apples, apricots, walnuts.

Silicon: Cucumbers, lettuce, parsnips, asparagus tips (raw), beet tops, dandelion, horseradish, leeks, okra, parsley, green peppers, radishes, spinach, watercress, strawberries, cherries, apricots, apples, watermelon, figs.

Iodine: Kelp, sea lettuce, carrots, Irish moss, pineapple. (Note: Do not use medicated or liquid iodine as a food or drink.)

That Greasy Fat In the Frier Goes Into Your Body!

Constipation is another corollary of eating foods cooked in excessively heated fats and oils, oils which are frequently heated over and over again, as are oils in fast food establishments as well as restaurants.

If you eat fried foods, you make it impossible to completely nourish your body constructively. The overheated fat interferes with the function of the liver in the proper use of the atomic and molecular elements in your food.

Once you know that excessive heat completely destroys the value of any fat for nutritional purposes, you may want to do what we do, and that is to diligently and assiduously avoid eating any food which has been fried.

Fats are essential components of the cells and tissues of the body, but only when the fats are natural and have not been subjected to excessive heat. Unheated and unprocessed fats used for salad dressings (which you will find in the back of this book) are quickly and completely emulsified and oxidized when digested and assimilated by the body.

Natural fats are needed to act as lubricants for the intestinal tract, (as they are also needed for lubrication of the entire body). A person whose body is deficient in lubricating fat has great difficulty in expelling feces and waste from the body.

For energy value, fats furnish 125% more energy than either carbohydrates or proteins. Fats are also invaluable for maintaining the vitamin balance in the body, as they are important carriers of vitamins A, D, E and K, as these are all soluble in fat. If you want a well-balanced diet, you should take this into consideration and include the fats that Nature means for us to have.

Honey Is Sweet, But Fat Delivers the Heat

As a source of energy the sugar-carbohydrate of honey, for example, has the advantage of furnishing energy quickly. While the energy supplied by fats is slower in manifesting itself, fats have double the energy potential of carbohydrates and consequently have the advantage of producing twice the volume of heat and "burn" slowly. For this slower burning quality, fats are more suitable as a storage material and fuel reserve.

In the final analysis, one must realize that the body requires a certain amount of fat to enable the human mechanism to function smoothly. The body of a man weighing, say, between 125 and 130 pounds will contain about 12 to 14 pounds of fat if he is in a fairly healthy condition, while the body of a woman of similar weight will contain between 32 and 37 pounds of fat.

This fat is essential because it serves as a food reserve and forms the most efficient concentrated fuel, both for maintaining the normal temperature of the body and to furnish energy for the power to carry on its functions.

Try Some of Nature's Wholesome Fats

In nutrition, the proper selection and use of fats is very important. Fatty acids are found in all foods, but in higher amounts in meat and dairy products. However, there are plentiful supplies of foods with low saturated fatty acids, and a correspondingly higher quantity of foods with unsaturated fatty acids. All we need do is to select the correct vegetables, fruits, seeds, nuts and oils, and avoid or reduce the use of animal food, heavy fats and greases, particularly the manufactured grease products.

With this information as your guide you can choose your food intelligently and avoid eating food containing an excess of the saturated fatty acids with their correspondent excessive cholesterol. Be assured, though, that cholesterol is an unnecessary nightmare for far too many people who are fearful that a mouthful of fat will cause the rapid degeneration of their blood vessels. As a matter of fact, the body needs cholesterol.

Nature's Fats Aren't Greasy!

For your guidance I am listing some of the foods in which the unsaturated fatty acids considerably exceed the saturated fatty acid content.

The numbers after each item in the following list indicate how many times more the unsaturated fatty acids are present than the saturated fatty acids. Thus, for example, an avocado has 3½ times more unsaturated fatty acids than the saturated.

Avocado 3½	Almonds 11
Brazil nuts 4	Chickpeas 10
Black walnuts 15	English Walnuts 13
Eggs 2	Millet 2
Hickory nuts 11	Olive Oil 8
Oats 3½	Pumkin seed 4½

Pistachio nuts 8½   Safflower oil 11
Rice 4½   Whole wheat 5
Sunflower oil 8   Filberts or Hazel
Corn Meal 7½   nuts 18
Olives 8   Sesame seeds 7¼
Pecans 12

One Man's Meat Is Another Man's Poison

Let me state here my position on the eating of meat. Neither I nor my wife eat meat. I concluded long ago, through my studies, that if I wanted to have the health and longevity that Nature intended, I would consider the consumption of meat a serious deterrent to her work.

I might also add (and I have discussed the subject later on) that I am not what many people would call a vegetarian. Vegetarians cook their vegetables, usually do not drink fresh, raw unprocessed vegetable and fruit juices, and eat cooked starches. While I am sure there must be many strict vegetarians, those who abstain from meat and dairy products, there are fewer who eat Nature's perfect diet. Man does not yet realize that Nature has a diet that will provide him with astoundingly good health, a weight that was tailored for his body, and a longer life expectancy.

Strange How Much You Have to Know
Before You Know How Little You Know

I have found that if a person has studied and informed himself (or herself) of the reasons for giving up a certain food, it is a powerful motivation to abstain permanently.

The eating of flesh is a custom handed down to this generation from thousands of years of a practice that has no foundation in reason. Man's taste for the flesh of animals is a tradition, and if he does not stop to ask whether or not it aids his health and longevity, he eats it and eventually may suffer the penalty for so doing.

Physiologically, the eating of meat increases the acidity of the body. In the process of digestion and the breaking down of the meat into its original amino acids, a vast amount of uric acid is generated in the body. If the body could eliminate this immediately, it might do only little harm. But, because the digestion is slow, the muscles absorb enormous amounts of uric acid, and in the course of time, they are saturated with it. Eventually this acid forms into crystals with sharp, needle-like points, which cause the pain and discomfort known as rheumatism, neuritis, sciatica, nephritis (Bright's disease), and some of the diseases of the liver.

In all my experience I have never found one individual who had lived on fresh, raw vegetables and fruits, and used an intelligent amount of fresh vegetable and fruit juices, for periods of five or ten years or more, who during that period had ever suffered with any of the ailments caused by the accumulation of uric acid in the body.

On the other hand, every case without exception that I have had contact with, where I have been able to check the person's diet, where the individual suffered from rheumatism, neuritis or sciatica, meat was invariably a regular part of the diet.

In the course of our research we have made thousands of analyses of urine, and, without exception, found that the urea present in the urine of meat eaters was only one-tenth to one-fifth of what should have been eliminated, indicating that the muscles were absorbing from five to ten times what the body should eliminate through the kidneys.

If for no other reason, one should refrain from eating meat or meat products, because of a desire to avoid the aches and ailments resulting sooner or later from the accumulation of uric acid in the system.

Your Big Juicy Steak Is Tainted with
Adrenalin Poison, Bacteria and Decay

When an animal is led to be slaughtered, it is filled with terror, just as any human being would be in its place. The animal's adrenal glands pour out so much adrenalin that the animal's body becomes tainted with it and remains so right up to the time man eats it. Within a few minutes after death every cell and tissue in the animal's body begins to disintegrate.

You should by now understand how powerful a poison adrenalin is when it gets out of control. When we, ourselves, become angry or filled with fear, this gland becomes more active than normal and more adrenalin flows into the blood, depending on the degree of fear or anger.

Habit Is Powerful and Custom Can Kill!

Because of man's habit of eating devitalized foods and existing in spite of them, it is difficult to convince people that the atoms in our foods must be live, organic atoms if we hope or expect to build for ourselves a vital body, free from sickness and disease. The lifeless, inorganic atoms in cooked and processed foods, by their very nature, cause the degeneration and disintegration of the body long before its time.

Just as life is dynamic, magnetic and organic, so is death static, non-magnetic, and inorganic. It takes life to beget life, and this applies to the atoms in our foods. When the atoms in amino acids are live, organic atoms, they can function efficiently. When they are destroyed by the killing of an animal or the cooking of food, the vital factors of the amino acids are lost!

Animals build larger, huskier and healthier bodies from the amino acids obtained from vegetation than man does by eating meat.

If more proof were needed to refute the farcical claims in favor of meat eating, we could look around for carnivorous animals to be suitable as beasts of burden and find none because they lack both the power and endurance. Herbivorous animals, however, from the horse, the oxen to the elephant all have phenomenal strength and endurance obtained from eating raw vegetation.

Of course I am not demanding that anyone's eating or living habits be changed. Each has the right to eat and live as he chooses. All I can do is point the way, and, let me remind you, I had to learn it the hard way.

Chapter 9
MAN'S ARTIFICIAL BEVERAGES

First, Let's Look At Nature's "Beverage."

The constitution of the human body consists of 56% to 70% water. One gallon of water is eliminated from the body every twenty-four hours through the pores of the skin, the kidneys and other eliminative organs. In order to maintain a correct, healthy water-balance, this loss of water must be replenished.

About one gallon of the water in the body is a component of the blood and circulates under pressure by the pumping action of the heart. By means of this pressure, the blood-water percolates through the tiny blood capillaries and permeates the space between the cells and tissues of the body, bathing every cell in the system with water. This blood-water is known as lymph, and circulates throughout the body through its own circulatory channels, which is known as the lymph system.

Nature Fights Back...

Whatever beverage you put into your mouth to drink goes into the blood first. Then the lymphatic system extracts any toxins. Furthermore, the lymph also collects noxious material and bacteria anywhere in your system in order to prevent their entering into the blood stream.

But Sometimes She Loses

When the lymphatic system has reached the point of tolerance for toxic and noxious liquids, the lymph glands become engorged. The final product of such engorgement may be tumors, cancer, elephantiasis, Hodgkin's disease, leukemia and other ailments in which such engorgement is a contributing factor. It is therefore very well worthwhile to resist putting toxic liquids into our bodies.

Your Soft Drinks Are Drugged

Soft drinks do not belong in the healthy human system, much less in an overweight body! Do you have any idea of what enters into the manufacturing of soft drinks? Sugar, first of all, "pure white sugar," which is a man-made drug, and should be called so. Phosphoric acid, a corrosive ingredient, is used in the sugar-refining process. Carbon dioxide is used for the "fizz" in the product, and when you drink it, additional volumes of carbon dioxide are added to the superfluous volume of it in your body. (The additional volume of carbon dioxide also speeds up the heartbeat, a potential danger for those people with heart problems.) And finally, the coloring matter — often a coal tar product — is used to attract the eye and deceive the mind.

Nine Chemicals and Only One Calorie

Many "dieters" want to substitute "sugar free" soft drinks instead of those with white sugar which they formerly drank. Unfortunately, "sugar free" soft drinks are just as hazardous to your health as the regular kind, in fact, even more dangerous!

Supposing you knew that soft drinks could cause your brain to disintegrate, would you drink them?

If you knew that more than a million children today are afflicted with cerebral lesions caused by soft drinks, would you keep your children from drinking them?

If the labels on the cans and bottles of soft drinks were marked, "Poison!" wouldn't you stop buying them immediately — and warn your children of their danger?

What Webster Says About "Poison."

Let me share with you an analysis of the word "poison. " It has a broad interpretation: "Any agent which introduced into the organism may chemically produce an injurious or deadly effect. That which taints or destroys purity; to exert a baneful influence, to corrupt."

Artificial Colorings and Artificial Flavorings
Produce Artificial Children

I am not making a wild assertion when I say that by drinking beverages and eating foods which have been artificially colored and flavored, millions of school children are today suffering serious ailments.

These children, who are eating a "normal diet," suffer disturbances which result in difficulty in concentration, especially in the area of reading and spelling. Sometimes they exhibit compulsive behavior.

From a Sweet Little Angel to a Naughty Little Devil

I have a friend whose niece is afflicted with this ailment. When this little girl's diet is carefully supervised by her mother and her teachers at school, making sure she has no concentrated sweets and especially no foods with additives and artificial colorings, she is as sweet as an angel and a joy to be with. (In fact, children with this affliction generally become normal within a matter of two or three weeks after the diet has been changed.) On the other hand, when this "sweet little angel" returns to her old eating habits, usually in the summer months, when supervision is more difficult, her behavior is so loud, erratic and hyperactive, that she is impossible to be with. She cannot sit still long enough for anyone to engage her in conversation, and generally behaves as one possessed!

Thankfully, her diet usually keeps this situation under control, but she will have to be educated to understand how she must eat and drink when she is older.

To me this is proof of the great danger to anyone using artificially colored and flavored products, much less those containing sugar.

Soft Drinks — Soft Heads

It is incredible but true that more than 80% — that's right — more than eighty percent of the manufactured beverages and foods sold in supermarkets and fast food stores are compounded from chemicals using artificial colors and flavors to make them salable. How absurd it is to drink a beverage that is so distasteful it has to be dyed and artificially flavored to be appealing!

The potential danger in drinking these beverages is the possibility of a chemical reaction causing serious disturbances in the body. The greatest danger is when the brain area is afflicted by the chemical constituents of soft drinks.

Adults in offices and factories consistently drinking soft drinks are also liable to be afflicted to a lesser form of cerebral lesions than those experienced by a child. They feel a "lift" while imbibing these soft drinks and even for a short while after. Such an uplift is elusive, though, and the letdown results in fatigue, poor concentration, and, frequently, headaches.

How Would You Like Your Soft Drink?
Red, Blue or Green?

Let's take a look at a partial list of dyes and colorings listed as ingredients on bottles, cans and packets of soft drinks on market shelves:

Aniline Dyes: You will rarely find aniline dyes mentioned by their names. They are generally classified as "artificial coloring." Some of these dyes are very acid and you should become familiar with at least some of the worst. While such dyes affect the body adversely, their reaction may vary in different types of people.

Amaranth (red), **Bordeaux** (brown), **Orange I** (yellow) and **Ponceau** (scarlet): These are all derived from compounding nitrogen and benzene. **Benzene** is obtained from the distillation of coal. It is used as a motor fuel, as a solvent for resins and rubber, and in the manufacture of dyes. It is an ingredient in coloring beverages. As chemical compounds, these dyes are harmful because they afflict the nervous system and the cerebrospinal fluid.

Sodium Phosphate: Sodium phosphate occurs in the blood and in the urine. Artificially, it is used as a dye, a coloring agent and is used in weighting silk. It is also used as an artificial coloring for beverages. Like all chemically manufactured substances, sodium phosphates interfere with the normal, smooth functions of the endocrine glands, throwing the body out of balance.

Guinea Green (dark green): This is a dye obtained by the reaction of chloroform with benzene and aluminum chloride. Chloroform has a sweetish taste. It is used as an anesthetic to put people to sleep. It produces violent gastroenteritis, which is an inflammation of the bowel and of the stomach. It results in complete unconsciousness when taken alone internally. Aluminum chloride is derived from heating aluminum with chlorine. It is used in oil refineries for "cracking" oils. The effect of aluminum on the body manifests in neuralgia, loss of energy, constipation, skin troubles, nausea, loss of appetite and many other afflictions.

Naphthol (yellow): This dye is compounded by nitrogen and benzene extracted from coal and is a coal tar product. Coal tar products can have very serious and harmful effects on the system.

Tartrazine (yellow): This is obtained by the action of acetylene on diazomethane, producing a poisonous chemical which is nevertheless used as a coloring agent in beverages and foods. This word, "poisonous" should warn you.

Whenever you read "Artificial Coloring" on a label, remember that there is no indication whatever which dyes are used for this purpose. It could be any one or a combination of these.

"I'll Have the Chemical Flavor Please."

As is the case with the use of artificial colors, there are innumerable substances used to give beverages and foods a flavor as nearly as possible to that of the fruit flavor they try to imitate. This product may not have been within miles of the fruit imitated, so artificial compounds are added to make the product palatable. The following list is but a small sampling of the imitation flavors used in soft drinks:

Caramel: This is obtained by heating sugar to more than 350°F, or by using ammonia with molasses or glucose. Besides using caramel as a red-yellow coloring agent, it adds a sugary zest to the flavor. The use of caramel tends to throw the blood out of balance, causing heart trouble which is intensified by the presence of ammonia. When used in excessive amounts, it can cause mental and other disorders, particularly with children.

Citric Acid: In citrus fruits citric acid is present in live, organic form, in which state it is beneficial as a alkalinizing beverage.

When citric acid is made chemically, however, and used in soft drinks, it increases the negative acidity of the system. If the organic citric acid were used in soft drinks it would tend to make the price almost prohibitive, whereas it can be made chemically very cheaply. Such chemical citric acid can cause canker sores in the mouth, and even ulcers in the duodenum.

Potassium Phosphate: This is also an acid component for fertilizers. It is also used in soft drinks with carbonated water to effervesce, or "fiz" the beverage.

Sodium Citrate: This is used as a prescription for certain genitourinary (genital urinary) disease. It, too, is added to soft drinks to give them a citric "zip."

Would You Enjoy Some Mexican Lice in Your Soft Drink?

Cochineal: This is a dye consisting of the dried bodies of lice which feed on cacti in Mexico and other parts of central and South America. Special cacti are extensively cultivated for the express purpose of propagating the cochineal lice. The female louse is gathered and killed by heat, then dried and pulverized. It yields a bright castillian red. It is rarely if ever mentioned as cochineal but may find its way into almost any product as "artificial coloring." It is also known as quillaja.

Coca: Coca is a South American and African nut containing 2% caffeine, theobromine and tannin. It is analogous to coffee. In normal doses it stimulates the brain, causing nervous restlessness and wakefulness. In larger doses it produces insomnia, paralysis of the heart muscles, convulsions, delirium, and other afflictions.

Cola: Cola is a plant grown throughout South America and in India. It is the derivative of cocaine, causing stimulation of the brain, resulting in normal sex desires being inhibited, it increases heart action and the irritability of the nerves, followed by mental, and muscular depression. It deadens the sensation of hunger and thirst temporarily but greatly increases these when the effects wear off. It gives a temporary sense of hilarity and well-being. Eventually the individual may look haggard and worn-out.

Man Against Himself

The question of why supposedly intelligent people imbibe soft drinks has puzzled me for a very long time. Could it be a quirk in the human mind that would keep people from being individualistic enough to stop putting something in their bodies which would cause eventual suffering? Or, could it be that they are not aware of the ultimate destruction which they are building up in their bodies?

If you want to give Nature a chance to improve your body, within and without, you will heed her warnings on the labels of man's artificial foods and beverages. When we give Nature the implements to work with, and submit ourselves without reservation to her ministrations, she will not let us down. She may find more things to correct in our bodies than we have any idea of, but if we will trust her to correct everything in turn, she will do a marvelous job for us and she will keep us slim and healthy.

Chapter 10
BEER AND OTHER ALCOHOLIC BEVERAGES
The Beer Unfit for a King

According to archeological discoveries, beer made from cereals has been used for some six thousand years. It was made from the fermentation of cereals to obtain the alcoholic effect.

It is recorded that about five thousand years ago, in the year 3000 B.C., in Egypt, four types of beer were made from grains grown in that country. The Pharaohs paid their peasants four loaves of bread and two jugs of beer as recompense for their labor, instead of paying them money.

Somewhat more recently, in 1200 B.C., the Pharaoh Rameses boasted of having contributed 465,000 jugs of beer to his pagan deities.

Through the centuries, cereals were grown to a great extent for making beer by the process of fermentation. Barley, wheat and oats were the most commonly used. For flavor, hops were added occasionally forty to fifty centuries ago.

Beer Is Big Business — But Who Profits?

The production of beer in the United States of America exceeds 3,875,000,000, yes, more than 3¾ billion gallons a year. The British and German workingmen consider beer and ale their heritage. Britain has the highest rate of kidney degeneration among civilized countries, except Germany. The U.S.A. is fast catching up with these countries.

Beer: Fascinating but Deadly

Beer has a peculiar fascination for nearly everyone who drinks it habitually. The average alcohol content of beer ranges between only 3% to 5%. The low alcoholic content of beer does not have an immediate reaction like that of a cocktail or of drinking straight potions like whiskey, vodka, champagne and the like. It is generally assumed that, because of the low alcoholic content, beer is an innocuous beverage. This is a very deceptive assumption, because, beer drinking actually results in a long-range degenerative reaction.

Beer making requires such hard water that the manufacturers frequently have to add as much as thirty-five times more minerals than are present in the water supply, using vast quantities of gypsum. Gypsum is a calcium-sulfate used for making plaster of paris. The use of gypsum is for increasing the calcium content of the water. And people drink beer without the knowledge or the thought of the plaster of paris they are drinking.

Beer is probably the most destructive liquid which we can put into our system. I have examined a tremendous number of kidneys at autopsies, and I could invariably determine correctly the alcoholic habits of the deceased.

On a Hot Day There's Nothing Like a Can of Barley Fermented with Yeast and Flavored with Hops!

The alcohol in beer is much more subtle in its harmful effects than are other alcoholic beverages. The period which elapses between drinking a glass of beer and its reaction on the body involves the element of time, because of the three-phase affect:

The first phase is a period of excitement and of entrancement which gratifies and seduces the sense organs and transmits the stimulation to the nerve centers.

In the second phase, the low alcoholic content is just enough to create an activity of excitement in the midriff, which is the center of the system, the region of the solar plexus. This activity is insidiously dangerous because there is nothing to counteract it.

In the third phase, the hops in the beer have an unhealthy reaction on the system. The hops used in making beer are used for the purpose of adding flavor and an extra tingle. Not many people, apparently, are aware of the noxious effect of hops on health. The damage, which results from the calcium and other mineral elements in the water as a clogging medium, interferes with the blood circulation, and is aggravated by the evanescent uplift of the low alcoholic content of the beer.

From a health standpoint, while hops are used medicinally as a tonic and a stimulant, they also affect the nerves, creating a loss of sensation. Hops also have an hypnotic effect and could cause delirium tremens, the same violent delirium tremens induced by alcohol. Other afflictions resulting in the use of hops can be hysteria, nervous insomnia, dyspepsia, rheumatism, and irritation of the bladder.

It seems hardly necessary, after discussing the rather gruesome effects beer has on the body, to add that beer makes you fat!

Alcohol's First Stop — The Brain!

The average alcoholic content of wines is in the neighborhood of 15%. Hard liquor contains a disastrously high percentage of alcohol, which causes the drinker to behave in a manner which is inverse to his natural self.

The most damaging alcoholic evil is the affliction which these beverages cause to the human brain. Alcohol is the only substance which can pass through the walls of the stomach directly into the bloodstream. It is picked up by the blood and transported quickly to the brain areas. The most important and the most vital, sensitive impulses, functions and activities of the body are generated in the brain. That is the reason one's actions are unpredictable once an alcoholic drink has slipped down the throat.

There are many cells in the human body which are composed of elements that are either only soluble in alcohol, or are dangerously afflicted by it. As an example, consider the crystalline sugar which is analogous to glucose, present in the brain tissues and known as cerebrose. This substance is quickly affected by alcohol. It is closely involved in the cerebrospinal fluid which, through the hypothalamus in the midbrain regulates the eyes, the ears and the individual's equilibrium or balance. (You can readily see why bleary-eyes, uncertain hearing and wobbly walking are indications of having indulged in alcohol.) When this cerebrose substance dissolves and appears in the urine it indicates the serious condition known as cerebral diabetes.

Of all the beverages best left alone, alcoholic beverages are number one.

Chapter 11
MILK AND DAIRY PRODUCTS
Some Illusions About Milk

It is generally assumed that cow's milk is one of our most perfect foods.

This half-truth is more misleading than a deliberate lie! Milk is the most mucous-forming food in the human diet, and, from infancy to senility, it is the most insidious cause of colds, flu, bronchial troubles, asthma, hay fever, pneumonia, tuberculosis and sinus trouble, according to our experience. It is almost superfluous to add that milk consumed by the adult or the child results in the condition we all know as overweight!

Cow's Milk Is for the Calf!

Milk is intended as food for the young, from birth until the skeletal bones and the rest of the anatomy are sufficiently developed for the assimilation of the natural foods required by the animal concerned. Thus, cow's milk was never intended for a human infant. Nature meant it as nourishment for the calf!

A child's nutrition is natural when it is provided from its mother's milk. Such milk contains water, natural sugars, salts, amino acids, hormones, vitamins, and the atoms of the elements necessary for the growth of the little body. One of the most important elements in milk is a substance called casein, which furnishes a vast number of amino acids for the construction of the protein molecules building up the child's body.

Cow's milk is vastly coarser than mother's milk, and it contains 300% more casein than human milk. Cow's milk is intended to double the weight of the calf in six to eight weeks, whereas a child's body requires six to seven months to double its weight. Cow's milk builds up the body structure of the calf to attain a weight of one thousand to two thousand pounds at maturity. I have yet failed to find a man or woman whose ambition is the attainment of even 250 or 300 pounds of weight!

The vast percentage of casein in cow's milk, however, is not digested and assimilated constructively by the human body. Except in rare cases, cow's milk is useless as human food.

The need for cow's milk as a necessary part of the human diet is purely and simply advertising propaganda with no foundation in fact. The recommendation of its use by any member of the healing profession is indicative of a lack of knowledge of the simple laws of the physiology of nutrition, and a lack of perception as to the fundamental cause of excessive mucus in the system.

There is not a member of the animal kingdom which uses milk as food after it has been weaned. It remains for man to develop such stupidity and to overlook the use of milk as the cause of so many of his ailments.

Nature placed the necessary ingredients in the milk of each type of animal best suited for the growth of its young.

Pasteurization

I will suffice it to say that the pasteurization of milk is no safeguard whatsoever for the health of the individual or of the community, and that it only prevents the milk from souring.

The claim that raw milk causes undulant fever and other diseases which would be prevented if it were pasteurized, is an utter and unmitigated falsehood. Pasteurization does not kill typhoid germs, nor bacilli coli, nor the germs of tuberculosis or of undulant fever.

In order to kill these pathogenic germs the milk would have to be heated to a temperature ranging all the way from 190°F. to 230°F.!

Propaganda and miseducation has caused the majority of people to use pasteurized cow's milk as food in the belief that it is a complete food for humans of all ages from the cradle to the grave.

Cream: A Superb Substitute for Milk

While milk is a concentrated food because it comes from an animal and contains complete protein and amino acids suited to the cow's body, cream is a fat and its digestion is entirely different. While, of course, it is somewhat mucous-forming, it is nevertheless a fairly good fat.

Cream should be used raw, not pasteurized, and in reasonable amounts. We find it particularly delicious when used on bananas sweetened with honey as a most satisfying breakfast. We also use it in many salad recipes, which you will find in the back of this book.

The Big, Big, Big Cheese!

I mention cheese here because, while it is certainly not a beverage, it comes from cow's milk, and most "dieters" want to know if cheese can be a part of their diet, as it is a filling and satisfying food.

The stronger the cheese, the greater is its acidforming effect on the body, and the more mucousforming it is. Cottage cheese (preferably the homemade kind) is probably the least mucous-forming, while seasoned Swiss cheese, the kind that is made in huge, round pieces about three feet across and eight or ten inches thick, with large holes all through it, is the next best cheese product to be a part of the diet.

When Tempted,
Don't Forget the Buttermilk Lady!

As a beverage, buttermilk does not have any particular virtue as nourishment. I have found none that I can consider to be of any particular benefit to the human body.

I was amused to see and hear a demonstration of cultured buttermilk at a health lecture some time ago. The lady demonstrating it was not the least bit bashful in boasting about the benefits she was deriving from drinking it three times a day. Nevertheless, I do not suppose it ever occurred to her that during the years she said she had been using it, flabby, excessive adipose tissues had accumulated to an almost alarming extent.

Her contour had the beautiful conformation of a flour sack tied in the middle, and her dripping nose required a constant flourish of a large handkerchief. This is what we mean when we say that diary products are mucous-forming.

The Art of the Herbalist — Revived!

There are thousands of herbs available to man. There is a revival of interest in herbs, both as beverages and for their healing qualities. As a result, there are now many, many varieties of herb teas on the market. Their value is inestimable.

If you want to drink the herb teas hot, they should not be boiled, but steeped in hot water at a temperature of not much over 125°F., in order to obtain the maximum benefit from them. You will also find that cold herb teas are quite refreshing on a hot day.

The truly constructive beverages are those which are replete with enzymes, and there are ample choices in fresh, uncooked, unprocessed vegetable and fruit juices, and herb teas. Water, of course, is an excellent beverage if it is distilled. The question of water is a subject that anyone who is serious about what beverages they put into their mouth should study carefully. As it would take too much space here to discuss the subject of water, I will refer you to my book on water, *Water Can Undermine Your Health.*

Let Nature Help You Out of Your Dilemma!

In the final analysis, we can get all the nourishment that we perhaps thought was provided in milk by turning to Nature. She will provide the most nourishing and refreshing beverages from fresh, raw vegetables and fruits, which are replete with all the mineral and chemical elements, vitamins, hormones and amino acids we need.

If the juices are properly made, fresh, from good quality vegetables, one can obtain plenty of proteins, carbohydrates and natural sugars. In addition, fresh fruits and vegetables are rich in calcium and all the other minerals necessary for good health. Among the richest calcium foods are carrot, turnips, spinach and dates.

If this is the first time you have ever read about what Nature intends for you to eat, you may well wonder why other people, including yourself, are not eating this way.

I learned years ago that all people are not ready for Nature's diet. Mankind's traditions are stronger than the good, common sense that is found in Nature's laws. People choose their foods and their pleasures according to their state of awareness. People whose state of awareness is that of the mass instinct will consider this diet as being crazy. Anything that is out of the ordinary, and which is beyond their understanding is an anathema, idiotic — not withstanding all proof to the contrary.

When a person has risen to a higher state of awareness, whether by accident or by design, they will find that they need food of a higher vibration than the dead, cooked and processed foods that human tradition demands.

At this point, let me encourage you in your quest for better health and the body weight only Nature can give you, by assuring you that you are on the right track. As for the "how to's," of being able to make these fresh fruit and vegetable juices in your own kitchen, and of making delicious uncooked meals for yourself or for your whole family, I can assure you that every help I can possibly give you will be included in these pages.

Bearing in mind all I have related in this chapter, I have but one thing more to say to you: "Think before you drink"!

Chapter 12
PROTEIN

A Word About Vegetarians

When people who do not know my eating habits learn that I do not eat any meat, fish or fowl, they ask, "Where, do you get your protein?"

I think this is one of the questions most frequently raised when the matter of vegetarianism is discussed. It shows how vast the lack of knowledge is concerning the rebuilding of the cells and tissues of the body. It also proves that people have no conception of the effect that the digestion of concentrated protein, which we have already discussed, has on the health and longevity of the body.

It is oftentimes remarked that vegetarians as a rule are not particularly good examples of health and vitality. Would it surprise you if I said that I agree with this criticism? If not, then you are learning why Nature's diet is unique!

The vegetarians whose bodies betray minimum standards of health and vitality, are those who have merely eliminated meat from their diets. They consume vast quantities of cooked grain and starchy foods. They do not eliminate sugar from their diets and, often, they cook all or most of their vegetables! They do not drink enough, if any, fresh vegetable or fruit juices. On such a diet it is virtually impossible to have a healthy body, much less a slim one.

The True Vegetarian Defined

Under the circumstances, it is not really right to judge vegetarians as a class, unless the classification is defined. Strict, raw food vegetarians, who drink plenty of fresh vegetable and fruit juices, who avoid cooking their grains and other foods, and eschew meats of all kinds, are, without exception, outstanding individuals who have healthy, trim bodies, bursting with good spirits and vitality — particularly if they were brought up from childhood to shun and avoid these foods. This is not by any manner or means fanatical. It is just plain common sense and perfectly natural proven without question from experience!

Please! Don't Eat "Fake Meat."

A word of warning to those who use soy "meat" substitutes! When soy substitutes are ingested, the protein-digestive juices are alerted to care for concentrated proteins, as the mind vicariously enjoys the flavor of meat. There being no concentrated protein present, these protein-digestive juices "attack" the "substitute," which is usually compounded from cooked grains, soy beans and starches. The result is the indigestibility of the food with repercussions of toxemia as the end-product.

Protein Is Abundantly Available

Where do I get my protein from? The most constructive protein is available in fresh, raw vegetable juices. The combination of carrot-celery-parsley-and spinach juices, classified as "potassium juice," is one of the richest sources of protein. This combination of juices is the most easily digested and assimilated in the vegetable juice family.

The juices of Brussels sprouts, savoy cabbage, collards, dandelion, kohlrabi, lettuce, parsley, salsify, spinach, turnips, all have individually a very high protein content. Such juices should always be taken with some carrot juice in their combinations. If some of these vegetables are unfamiliar to you, it just may be that you haven't noticed them in your market. Most are not hard to obtain, and the juice combination recipes included in this book will take away the mystery about them.

Proteins are the main constituents of the cells and tissues of the body, and are composed of about twenty-three variations of amino acids. No protein, nor any of the amino acids, enter the liver, as such, but must be broken down by the digestive process into the atoms and molecules composing them. Then the processing by the liver reassembles and converts the atoms and molecules into such amino acids and proteins as are needed for the body's regeneration.

Protein Shows Up in the Most Surprising Places

There are three sources from which the liver receives material for the body's reconstruction of needed amino acids and protein, namely:

1. From the protein content of vegetables, fruits, nuts and seeds, and from fresh, raw vegetable and fruit juices.

2. From the concentrated protein of the flesh of animals, fish and fowl, and from concentrated "food supplements."

3. From the air we breathe!

The third source, air, is not generally perceived as necessary protein nourishment. The air we breathe is 79% nitrogen and 21% oxygen. Nitrogen is an essential constituent of all the amino acids and proteins!

The nitrogen in the air we breathe is gathered from the lungs by the blood and delivered to the liver. It is converted by the liver into the atomic ingredients for the reconstruction of amino acids with which to build cell proteins.

Once again, Nature provides a simple source for the body's needs. She has provided those elements from the air that surrounds us. All we need do is get out in the air, where it's fresh and clean, and take a walk. We will come back feeling refreshed, both in mind and spirit!

A Quick Course In Chemistry

Amino acids are compound elements composed of carbon, hydrogen, oxygen and nitrogen grouped into different patterns and in certain proportions.

To give a non-technical description of amino acids we could use the example of the many varieties of roses. As the colors, the petals and the patterns determine the type and variety of roses, so these groups of atoms determine the type and variety of amino acids. The amino acids, in turn, group into patterns which form the different kinds of flesh proteins.

If you are interested in the twenty-three amino acids, without which your body could not regenerate itself, you will find a complete list of them in my book, *Diet and Salad.* There is simply not enough room in this book to include this information, but if you should get a copy, you will find that it is particularly helpful in showing what each amino acid does in the body, and the food sources for each.

Here is a little sample of my amino acid list for you to see whether it would be helpful to you:

1. **Alanine:** Composed of 40% carbon, 8% hydrogen, 36% oxygen and 16% nitrogen.

Alanine's molecular weight is about 89. It is a component of calcium pantothenic acid (from the vitamin class) involved in the healthy condition of the skin, particularly that of the scalp and hair. It is also a factor in the balance and healthy operation of the adrenal glands.

The following raw foods contain alanine: alfalfa; raw, unsalted almonds; avocados; olives; cream; carrots; celery; dandelions; lettuce; cucumbers; turnips; green peppers; spinach; watercress; apples; apricots; grapes; oranges; strawberries; tomatoes.

Most people, who are not conscious of what foods they eat, are amazed to see how Nature's law of supply and demand is fulfilled by fruits and vegetables!

How much protein do we need a day? An adult does not need as much protein in proportion to weight as a child does. An infant requires a great deal more protein during the first and second years of life.

The relative use of protein building blocks in the child is greater because the body is in the process of growing and developing. The protein requirement of the adult is more constant and is limited chiefly to maintenance and replacement.

Meat: What Needless Harm It Brings Us

I have found in the course of my research, and in the studies of many other researchers, that the eating of meat increases the acidity of the body. As the process of digestion breaks the meat down into its original amino acids, a vast amount of uric acid is generated. If the body could eliminate this acid immediately, it might do only a little harm. But the body cannot quickly eliminate uric acid, and the muscles absorb enormous amounts of it!

In the course of time, the muscles become saturated with uric acid crystals which have sharp, needle-like points. Needless to say, pain and discomfort follows. Uric acid crystals within the muscles cause rheumatism, neuritis, sciatica, nephritis (Bright's Disease), and some of the diseases of the liver.

If for no other reason, we should refrain from eating meat or meat products to avoid the aches and ailments resulting, sooner or later, from the accumulation of uric acid in the system.

The eating of meat, then, is purely a matter of personal taste, preference and judgment. It is very definitely not a matter of supplying the body with necessary protein.

The eating of flesh is a custom handed down from generation to generation for thousands of years. As a practice, it has no foundation of need. Man's taste for the flesh of animals is a tradition, and without attempting to reason whether its use is constructive or destructive, he eats it, and may suffer the penalty for doing so.

Chapter 13
JUICES AND JUICERS
The Clue That Opened Up Nature's Secrets

My extensive studies in the healing arts gave me a clue, and this was many years ago, which led me to the discovery of the steps necessary to develop the kind of health I knew the body to be capable of, and an easy, natural way to maintain proper body weight. This clue, based on my earlier experiences with the healing and body-building ability of fresh carrot juice, led me to examine the body's digestion of all vegetable and fruit juices.

When we eat solid food, it must be broken down by the digestive system into liquids. This is necessary in order to separate the atoms and molecules from the food fibers so that they can pass through the walls of the intestine, where they are picked up by the blood stream and delivered to the liver.

Due to these studies, I found that fresh, raw juices relieve the digestive system of much of the energy required to liquify solid food. More importantly, while solid food takes three to five hours to digest, juices are digested in a matter of minutes, and they are assimilated into the system in a very few minutes more.

Now, do not jump to the conclusion that we should live solely on juices, eating no solid food. We do need to eat plenty of fresh, raw solid food, in the form of vegetables, fruits, nuts, seeds and their sprouts. The fibers of these solid foods are needed as roughage, in order to act as an intestinal broom, figuratively speaking, so that the colon can have fibrous material to assist its movement in expelling the waste products from the body.

On the other hand, an entirely raw food regimen without the inclusion of a sufficient quantity and variety of fresh, raw juices is equally deficient. The reason for this deficiency lies in the fact that a surprisingly large percentage of the atoms making up the nourishment in raw foods is utilized as fuel for energy by the digestive organs. The atoms from the raw vegetables and fruits furnish some nourishment to the body, but for the most part are used up as fuel, leaving only a small percent for the regeneration of the cells and tissues.

An Apple a Day Cleans the Refuse Away

Fruit juices are the cleansers of the body. Fruits in sufficient variety will furnish the body with all the carbohydrates and sugar that it needs.

A Carrot a Day Keeps Illness At Bay

Vegetable juices are the builders and regenerators of the body. They contain all the amino acids, minerals, salts, enzymes and vitamins needed by the human body, provided they have been used fresh, raw and without preservatives, and have been property extracted from the vegetables.

A Dream Come True: the Juice Extractor

As I have earlier related, my first experiments with extracting the juices from carrots were made by grating carrots on anything that would reduce them to a pulp, then squeezing the pulp in a cloth to get the juice. After discovering the miracle of using that juice, so simply made, I tried making the carrots into a pulp by other means, until I could make a larger amount of juice for myself in less time and effort.

Eventually, I discovered a means to reduce the vegetables into fine particles, almost instantly into a pulp nearly as fine as apple butter, thereby splitting open the interstices (the small spaces) of the cells of the fibers, liberating the atoms and molecules. Then, by squeezing the pulp in a hydraulic press, I obtained a virtually complete extraction of the juice, and — it's quality was unsurpassed!

My interest and knack in developing mechanical contrivances, I achieved my objective — a complete, effective and efficient juicer extractor.

The manufacturers of this equipment wanted to perpetuate the recognition of my efforts in this discovery by putting my name on the label. As I objected to this, we compromised and they called it the first few letters of my name, the Norwalk Juicer, namely, NORman WALKer.

This company has been given the rights to use this name and to manufacture the machines on the condition that they would be made to last a lifetime, and so mechanically perfect that their efficiency and operation would require little or no service. Another condition was that the machines would be sold at the lowest price possible, consistent with the highest grade of material and workmanship.

Since the development of the Norwalk Triturator pulverizer and Hydraulic Press Juicer, many juicers of this centrifugal type have been developed, and there are some very satisfactory models on the market. The juicers of this centrifugal type have been used with benefit by many people. We need to drink juices daily, irrespective of how they are extracted. Any fresh juice is better than no juice at all.

The juice extracted by the centrifugal method should be used immediately, because unless the extraction of the juice from the fibers is as complete as it is humanly and mechanically possible to achieve, oxidation and heat from the friction will tend to spoil the juice in a short time.

Think Before You Drink

It hardly seems necessary, but I want to remind you again that all the juices must be raw. If they are canned, processed, preserved or pasteurized, their life principle has been destroyed and their vital value extinguished. On the other hand, the use of fresh, raw vegetable and fruit juices will supply the atoms and molecules needed to replenish the body. In addition, the drinking of these vegetables and fruits in their pristine state will provide you with the finest of organic water and all the organic chemical and mineral elements and vitamins possible to obtain.

How Do You Become a Juice Fan? Try It!

I have found that one can drink, with much benefit, several pints of fresh, raw vegetable juice daily, when properly made. One pint a day seems to be the least that will show perceptible results. Any discomfort from drinking them is usually due to the stirring up of conditions in the body which Nature is anxious to clear up, and, as soon as eliminated, an increase in vigor and energy will follow.

Just how much juices can be drunk every day would also depend on the condition of the individual. Raw carrot juice may be taken indefinitely in any reasonable quantities — from one to six or eight pints a day. It has the effect of helping to normalize the entire system, and in the case of one who is beginning a weight-loss program, this is a necessary step.

Just a Few of the Remarkable
Benefits of Carrot Juice

Carrot juice has the richest source of vitamin A, which the body can quickly assimilate. It contains also an ample supply of vitamins B, C, D, E, and K.

Raw carrot juice is a natural solvent for ulcerous and cancerous conditions. It's a resistant to infections, doing most efficient work in conjunction with the adrenal glands. It helps prevent infections of the eyes and throat as well as the tonsils and sinuses and the respiratory organs generally. It also protects the nervous system, and is unequalled for increasing body tone and vigor.

The Carrot: Nature's Method Of Cleaning House

Intestinal and liver diseases are sometimes due to a lack of certain elements which are found in properly prepared carrot juice. When these elements are provided by the drinking of carrot juice, a noticeable cleaning up of the liver may take place, and the material which was clogging it will be found to dissolve.

In some instances these toxins are released from the liver so abundantly that the intestinal and urinary channels are inadequate to care for this overflow, and in a perfectly natural manner they are passed into the lymph for elimination from the body by means of the pores of the skin. This material has a slightly yellow-orange tinge, not unlike a sun tan, and while it is being so eliminated from the body, it will discolor the skin. It is not the carrot juice itself, nor the carotene that comes through the skin, as this discoloration will take place even if the carrot juice is filtered to the point of clearing it of all color pigmentation.

Instead of becoming distressed over the possible appearance of skin discoloration, which will in any case disappear, we should be gratified that the disintegration of the liver has been stopped or prevented by the use of Nature's method of cleansing the body.

Aids to Help You On Your Way to Extraordinary Health and Permanent Weight-Loss.

In my book, *Fresh Vegetable and Fruit Juices,* I have discussed the various juices and their healing and regenerative properties. I have also included a list of ailments and the juice combinations which are beneficial to each condition.

For example,

Obesity:
Excessive adipose tissue resulting from incompatible combinations of foods and eating excessive quantities of starches and sugars....
Juices:
1. Carrot (as much as desired)
2. Carrot   10 oz.
    Spinach   6 oz.
3. Carrot   10 oz.
    Beet   3 oz.
    Cucumber   3 oz.

I have tried to provide as much material as possible in this book concerning the value of the various fruits and vegetables to certain health problems, as well as how they are prepared but space will not allow everything to be printed. However, for this book I have chosen that which I feel is most valuable and practical for one who is seeking to eat as Nature has provided.

In the back of this book, then, you will find many recipes in *Fresh Fruit and Raw Vegetable Salads.* Also included, a *Vegetable and Fruit Value Chart,* will be a practical help to you in determining just how much protein, carbohydrates, fats, and vitamins and minerals are in the fruits and vegetables you will be eating. Another section, *Fresh Fruit and Raw Vegetable Juice Drinks* lists the proportions of the various combinations of delectable and healthful juices.

Chapter 14
YOUR FIRST STEP
TOWARD A SLENDER, HEALTHY BODY

Your Insides Need a Housecleaning!

The very first procedure in achieving the weight that Nature meant you to have is a thorough cleansing of the colon by means of colon irrigations. If you are unfamiliar with this procedure, do not be discouraged. A colonic is a washing out of the colon, which is the large intestine in the body and the end process of digestion. It is simply a glorified enema, using many gallons of water — only a few ounces at a time - administered by a colonic operator. It is a method which involves a water flow and an explosion under the control of the operator, while the patient lies relaxed on an appropriate table which is connected with the colonic equipment.

To be efficient, a colon irrigation requires a period of half an hour to one hour. During that period, twenty to thirty gallons of water may have been inserted into the colon through the rectum, with the water flowing through the colon and then expelled each time.

Do You Know Your Body Has a Sewer?

The very purpose of the colon as an organ of elimination is to collect all fermentative and putrefactive toxic waste from every part of the anatomy, and, by the peristaltic waves of the muscles of the colon, remove all solid and semi-solid waste from the body.

In simple words, the colon is the sewage system of the body. Nature's laws of preservation and hygiene require that this sewage system be cleansed regularly, under penalty of innumerable ailments, sicknesses and diseases that follow, as the night follows the day, if waste is allowed to accumulate. Not to cleanse the colon is like having every garbage collector in your city go on strike for days on end. The accumulation of garbage in the streets would create putrid, odoriferous, unhealthy gases and be dispersed into the atmosphere.

Constipation: Nature's Early Warning Signal

The expression constipation is derived from the Latin word "constipatus," which translated means "to press or crowd together, to pack, to cram." Consequently, to be constipated means that the packed accumulation of feces in the bowel makes its evacuation difficult. However, a state of constipation can also exist when movements of the bowel may seem to be normal, in spite of an accumulation of feces somewhere along the line in the colon!

Constipation is the number one affliction underlying nearly every ailment. It can be imputed to be the initial, primary cause of nearly every disturbance of the human system. The most prevalent ailment afflicting civilized people is constipation. It is vital to stress that constipation affects the health of the colon, upon which the health of the body in its entirety depends.

There are two crimes against Nature which civilization indulges in as a daily routine, which beget this, the most common of our ailments, constipation. One is the consumption of devitalized and refined foods which fail to nourish the organs responsible for the evacuation of waste matter. The other, which is most prevalent particularly among young people, but not much less among the older and more mature, is neglecting to stop everything we are doing when the urge to evacuate the bowels should drive us headlong into the bathroom. Nature is a strict taskmaster: she gives one warning — sometimes two. You obey — or else! That "or else" is the insidious path to constipation.

Constipation Is Your Body's Greatest Enemy

If solving the problem of constipation were merely a case of washing out loose material lying free inside any part of the colon, it would not be too great a difficulty to clear the situation. An enema would most likely be sufficient to take care of its removal. The problem, however, is not quite so simple to dispose of. Constipation involves not only the unnecessary retention of feces in the bowel, but the retention is also present throughout the first half of the colon, from the cecum to the middle of the transverse colon. The cecum is located next to the ileo cecal valve at the beginning of the colon.

The wall of this section of the colon is equipped with sensitive nerves and muscles whose function it is to create peristaltic waves, to propel the contents of the colon from the cecum to the rectum for eventual evacuation. This is a distance of approximately five feet!

Things Are Seldom What They Seem!

If a person has eaten processed, fried and overcooked foods, devitalized starches, sugar and excessive amounts of salt, his colon cannot possibly be efficient, even if he should have a bowel movement two to three times a day! Instead of furnishing nourishment to the nerves, muscles, cells and tissues of the walls of the colon, such foods can actually cause starvation of the colon. A starved colon may let a lot of fecal matter pass through it, but it is unable to carry on the last of the digestive and nourishing processes and functions intended for it.

When the mineral elements which compose the foods we eat are saturated with oil or grease, the digestive organs cannot process them efficiently and they are passed out of the small intestine into the colon as debris. In addition, the body has a great deal of waste to dispose of through the colon in the form of used-up cells and tissues. When "demagnetized" food passes through the body system with little or no benefit, eventually, experience has proven that these foods leave a coating on the inner walls of the colon. In the course of time this coating may gradually increase its thickness until there is only a small hole through the center, and the matter so evacuated may contain much undigested food from which the body derives little or no benefit. The consequent result is a starvation of which we are not conscious but which causes old age and senility to race towards us with the throttle wide open.

What Do Pimples and Constipation Have In Common?

Obviously, if the feces in the colon have putrefied and fermented, any nutritional elements present in it would pass into the blood stream as polluted products. What would otherwise be nutritional becomes, in fact, the generation of toxemia.

Toxemia is a condition in which the blood contains poisonous products which are produced by the growth of pathogenic, or disease-producing, bacteria. Pimples, for example, are usually the first indication that toxemia has found its way into the body.

As the eliminative organs become afflicted with an accumulation of demagnetized and polluted products, the result is a constipated condition. The next best means of exit is through the pores of the skin and so we have pimples.

With this picture in mind, you can perhaps readily appreciate my claim that no system of dieting can be permanently effective until the eliminative organs have been cleansed,

A Lesson Learned by a Tragic Experience

Few of us realize that failure to effectively eliminate waste products from the body causes so much fermentation and putrefaction in the large intestine (the colon) that the neglected accumulation of such waste can, and frequently does, result in a lingering demise!

The reality of these colon facts was brought to my consciousness when I was a very young man. I was visiting my Aunt in Scotland when one morning a sudden piercing shriek was heard throughout the house from the living room. There, on the floor, curled up in a paroxysm of agony, was my favorite teen-age cousin. The doctor, who was immediately called, declared her appendix must have burst. She was rushed to the hospital in the family carriage, in the company of the doctor, but she died within a few hours. The old doctor said he did not know what caused the appendix to burst. He was not taught in medical school that is the natural result of neglecting the colon.

The kind and the quality of the food you put into your body is of vital importance to every phase of your existence. Good nutrition not only regenerates and rebuilds the cells and tissues which constitute your physical body, but also is involved in the processes by which the waste matter, the undigested food, is eliminated from your body to prevent corruption in the form of fermentation and putrefaction. This corruption, if retained and allowed to accumulate in the body, prevents any possibility of attaining any degree of health.

Fat, Pregnant or an Overloaded Colon?

As a matter of fact, we have seen that many people who have protruding stomachs were not suffering from an overweight condition at all. The shape of their contours were the result of failure to keep their colons cleansed of waste retention. The result of this waste matter accumulating in large amounts in the intestine reveals itself in an enlargement of the stomach.

Coupled with the failure to nourish the body with the proper foods, the retention of waste matter in the system results in the digestive and assimilative processes becoming overworked.

The Fate of a Gourmet

Many years ago, I was in business with a gentleman only a year or two older than I. He was a gourmand and an epicure — no food was quite sufficient enough for him. He ridiculed my way of eating and living, and we often had some strong discussions and arguments on the subject.

This gentleman's midriff advertised his way of living and eating — by the bulge! The very mention of cleansing the colon would spark his irascibility and his temper would flare up.

More than forty years ago, his death certificate read "Coronary Occlusion." The true verdict would have been "Intestinal Occlusion and Putrefaction." Anyway, he died much too young, while I, today forty years later, am alive, awake, alert and full of enthusiasm — thankful for Nature's teachings about the care of my body.

If you wish to further your studies about this important part of your body, the colon, I will refer you to my new book, *Colon Health: the Key to a Vibrant Life*.

If You're Serious, Get Going!

Based on several score years of experience, research and observation, it is my considered opinion that any mature man or woman who desires a long and healthy life, with a body weight that is best suited to them, should seriously consider their condition and take a series of colon irrigations and get started on this cleansing program.

How does one find a colonic operator? You can look in the yellow pages of your telephone directory for listings under Colonics or Colon Irrigations. Also call Chiropractors, Physiotherapists or Naturopaths and ask them if they employ colonic operators. You will have no trouble locating one.

It took many years for whatever corruption you may have to adhere to the inside walls of your colon; therefore, give the irrigations the chance to cleanse you thoroughly. Thereafter, I am convinced that about twice a year, throughout life, colon irrigations should help Nature keep the body healthy. Bear in mind that colon irrigations are far less expensive than hospitalization and surgical fees, and a better guarantee of beneficial results!

Chapter 15
YOUR SECOND STEP TOWARD
A SLENDER, HEALTHY BODY

Fast or Feast — What Shall It Be?

Instead of taking medication in order to reduce weight, it is far better to take the second step in Nature's diet by undertaking a controlled fasting program. Under no circumstances should one fast for more than six or seven consecutive days. The cleansing of the colon daily during a fast is a good idea if you can find a colonic operator or you can give yourself an enema. This cleansing prevents the reabsorption of toxins during the period that the body is undergoing cleansing. If such a period of fasting is not sufficient, then similar periods can be repeated after intervals of at least three or four days.

Bear in mind that a prolonged fast exceeding six or seven days will start a reverse process in the body. This means that the cells of the body will begin to feed on each other, lacking proper and natural nourishment. This could be very dangerous and may even become fatal. Fasting is very beneficial, but please do remember not to fast for any more than six or seven days at the utmost!

Give Your Digestive System a Holiday

During a fast no solid food should be eaten, but at least one gallon a day of good pure water or diluted fresh, raw fruit juices should be used as beverages, without fail. After a fast, no large quantities of solid food should be eaten for at least three to four days, as the body, having had the opportunity to rest from digestive labors and to relax, would rebel at so much sudden digestive activity. The best nourishment after a fast is the use of fresh raw vegetables and some fresh raw fruits for the following few days.

The effect of the fast is two-fold. It gives the digestive system and a great many other body functions a more or less complete rest. At the same time, it enables the body to burn up and eliminate waste. If you have never fasted before, you will be surprised at how your body will feel during its rest. You will not feel terribly uncomfortable. You must keep drinking the liquids though. To be careless about this will not bring the desired effect.

Your Body Will Thank You

As a general rule, I do not consider it advisable for most people to change their eating habits suddenly to a regimen of only raw foods. It seems to me that it is sometimes better to make the change gradually, yet as quickly as possible, consistent with the conditions of the individual.

When you have come off your fast and have begun eating small quantities of vegetables and fruits, I would suggest only eating raw foods for one, two or three days a week, and during the other days carefully planning the cooked meals so that every combination is absolutely compatible in accordance with the food combination chart in the back of this book. Also begin to drink one to two glasses of fresh, raw vegetable juices at the beginning of every meal, whenever possible. It should take but a short while to adapt one's self to the change.

It has been my experience that once the body has been thoroughly cleansed, and has become accustomed to such a regimen for several months or years, the individual becomes indefatigable, with an almost inexhaustible supply of energy, as well as a slim and trim body.

Put Your Faith in Nature's Table of Weights

Do not be mislead by the "Table of Weights" generally in vogue for dieting people. No two people are alike and the structure, height, in fact, the general build of the body should be the determining factor. You never see a race horse in training pulling a plough. Likewise, you never see a draft horse or a plow horse competing with race horses on the track. So it is with humans. Some people are overflowing with nervous tension and energy, while others are phlegmatic, if not downright lazy. It is a good thing that Nature provides her own "Table of Weights," for it is far more accurate than man could devise.

Throw Your Scales Out the Window!

It would only be human nature to keep an eye on your scale as the days of your fast pass by and the subsequent ones multiply. One of the most difficult facts to accept is that our body's timetable, just as our tables of weights, are not consistent with Nature's. Even though Nature takes her time, she will never let you down, nor will she ever harm your body. If you have been in the business of harming your body, then take some time to calculate just how much time Nature may have to take to regenerate it!

By the time Nature has done her job, your weight will be consistent with your body-build. If you continue Nature's diet, you will never have to stand on those weight scales again!

He Who Criticizes Is the Loser

When we embark on this program, which usually requires a complete change of our eating, drinking and living habits, we are nearly always confronted with the opposition of our family and friends. This is something we must learn to take in stride. To face and combat such opposition, we must have the courage of our convictions, based on the knowledge which we can acquire only through study and practice of the principles involved in this program.

We will always find more people ready to tear down and condemn, than to help and encourage. Once we have made a start and have begun to feel and express the surge of new life, energy and youthfulness, our assurance that we are on the right road should give us the means to combat any opposition.

Train Up a Child In the Way He Should Go and He Will Not Depart from It.

Let me add here at this point that this diet does not have to disrupt meal times within the family. As a matter of fact, all health begins at home. Our minds, especially the little children's, are fed on what we hear and see around us and what we are taught and what we read.

Until a child is old enough to start going to school, the parents are responsible for all the foods they set before their children and themselves. A child must not be permitted to grow up like a weed, with no special training in the home regarding morals, manners, self-discipline and respect for others' rights. Just as these things should be taught, parents must teach their children what to eat, and what not to eat.

Children have a tendency to want to imitate what others are doing, especially their parents. If they are served nutritious meals in the home, and taught why they must only eat what Nature provides, and see the example set before them by their parents, they will have healthy minds and healthy bodies.

As I look at older children today, teenagers, I find that they seem to be seeking a healthier diet and a better way of life. While I cannot speak for the majority, these young adults seem to be a very intelligent generation, searching for the truth wherever they can find it.

I have a friend whose children reacted in an amazingly positive way when their mother began to point out the ingredients in the foods at the supermarket where they shopped. These two teenagers, really young adults, supported their mother's decision to change their eating habits. Now, when they want something sweet, they blend their own concoctions of fruits in their juicer.

We Can Only Love Others If We First Love Ourselves

As we begin our fast and the cleansing of our body, bear in mind that to indulge our appetites and desires without regard to their final outcome may set us back every time. Wrong living and eating, without an intelligent purpose or aim will cause us sorrow and regrets later on. That is the question that every one of us must answer for himself, every time.

We cannot live for ourselves alone, although the "I" is the most important element in our existence. Unless we take care of ourselves first and foremost, we cannot be of any good or value to ourselves nor to anyone else. Therefore, our first consideration must begin with ourselves. The care and attention we give to our physical, mental and spiritual body will reflect our value to the rest of the world. If we neglect to care and develop our own trinity — our physical, mental and spiritual system — we will soon become useless to ourselves and to the rest of the world. We must feel proud of our physical bodies in both health and appearance.

Knowledge is like the seeds of plants. Keep them tucked away, and the seeds are eventually worthless. Plant, cultivate and nourish them. The whole neighborhood will gaze at and enjoy the splendor of your garden. This, in turn, will bring you more seeds, because you made good use of the first fruits of your labor.

Chapter 16
FOOD COMBINING
Your Body is a Food Processing Center

The manner in which our food is prepared by mastication and insalivation has considerable influence in the process of digestion and in the ultimate emission of the fiber and other non-digestible material from the small intestine into the colon. The finer the mastication, the easier is the work of the digestive glands and the liver.

Once the food gets into the stomach it is entirely cut off from any activity or passage through any part of the digestive system, except during the seconds when the pyloric valve opens to let a minimal amount of the liquefied bolus pass through at regular intervals. This allows the various gastric juices in the stomach to work on the specific type of mineral-chemical elements of which the food eaten was composed. There is a definite orderliness in the movement of the stomach, especially in the separation and ejection of the more liquid parts of the bolus from the more solid.

The dome of fundus of the stomach is not, as many suppose, to cushion air which is expelled when burping. It has been put there for the stomach to use as a storage place for retaining the bulk of food while the activity of the pylorus macerates the bolus and passes it out into the duodenum (small intestine) from time to time. The movement of the bolus starts within a few minutes after it has entered the stomach.

The stomach is flat and in a state of collapse until food is eaten. Then each subsequent mouthful takes its turn in being processed by the gastric juices between the cardiac sphincter and the pylorus. Carbohydrate foods pass from the stomach soon after ingestion and require only about half the time required by proteins for complete gastric processing. Fats, however, when eaten alone remain in the stomach a long time and when combined with other foods, their passage through the pylorus is considerably delayed.

Because of the chemical nature of both our bodies' digestive systems and of the foods we eat, it is vital that we understand how to eat proper combinations of foods so that the body can efficiently use them for good health and maintenance of body weight.

Orange Juice and Oatmeal Do Not Mix

In chemistry, oil and water do not mix, nor do acids mix with alkaline substances. They are totally incompatible. Such is the case with the food we eat. In the preparation of our meals, every food present represents a chemical combination of elements — atoms and molecules — according to the plan of Nature. When these foods are composed of raw vegetables and fruits, the elements composing them are vital, organic, live elements, and can be combined in any desired mixture. Any mixture that has not been cooked or processed can be eaten together because the elements combine in a natural manner and the result is beneficial to the body. When the foods are processed or cooked, however, the elements composing them have become devitalized. This applies to all of these foods, without exception.

Your Stomach Is Well-Organized — Unless You Put the Wrong Food In It!

Chemically, carbohydrates (sugars, starches and grains) are alkaline substances, and they need an alkaline digestive medium in the stomach for proper and complete processing. Proteins, on the other hand, are acid substances which require their own specific acid digestive juices.

When a carbohydrate enters the stomach it receives a disinfecting hydrochloric acid bath because the delicate lining of the intestine it will be later entering can be harmed by the presence of infectious elements. When a protein enters the stomach it also is disinfected by the hydrochloric acid, after which the protein digestive juice pepsin is secreted by the glands in the stomach, and the breaking down of the protein begins to take place.

Don't Put a Mass of Confusion Into Your Stomach

The natural sequence of this acid-alkaline chemical law is disrupted when we eat concentrated foods. If we eat an alkaline food, such as potatoes, and at the same time eat an acid one, such as chicken, the chicken is not properly digested because it is infiltrated by the acid and pepsin protein digestive juice. The meat (protein) is likewise interfered with by the presence of the carbohydrate in the chyme. The result of this incompatible condition is the fermentation of the carbohydrate and the putrefaction of the proteins.

The Road to Constipation Is Paved With Proteins and Carbohydrates

To make matters worse, if the protein was eaten before the carbohydrate, the passage of the carbohydrate out of the stomach will be retarded. When carbohydrate and protein foods of a concentrated nature are eaten together, the bolus of such a combination is treated first by the protein enzymes in the upper part of the stomach and the carbohydrate food is thereby "contaminated." When, at its allotted time, the bolus reaches the middle part of the stomach, further acidulation by hydrochloric acid takes place. The result of this delay causes the carbohydrate food to remain in the stomach longer than necessary for its own enzyme processing. This is likely to result in its eventual fermentation along its way to absorption and elimination. This condition can have a serious bearing on a person's elimination problems.

Eating the Wrong Foods Can Be Complicated
Eating Natural Foods Are Easy

It is an easy matter to remember the difference between the natural and the concentrated foods if we bear in mind that all vegetation contains both carbohydrates (in the form of natural sugars) and proteins in the form best suited for processing by human digestion. The concentrated carbohydrates and proteins require a greater amount of digestive processing, thus causing a great burden of labor on the digestive organs.

Here are some examples of concentrated carbohydrates and proteins, which should not only be avoided in combination, but avoided completely!

Bread with eggs or flesh food of any kind
Coffee and sugar
Hamburgers and soft drinks
Meat and potatoes with biscuits
Pie or cake with coffee or tea
Soups containing flour of any kind (for thickening) with meat
    stock or pieces of meat

Fruits and Vegetables — Nature's Best Combination

With few exceptions I have found that raw fruits and vegetables are perfectly compatible when eaten together, either mixed in a salad or separately during the same meal. Melons of all kinds, though, should be eaten alone, the whole meal consisting of nothing but melon. Melons require an unusual time to digest, thus you would be leaving whatever else you ate with the melon to sit in the stomach for much too long a time.

If You Have An Alkaline Stomach:

Fruits should only be eaten when they are ripe, because their sugars have not formed completely and therefore will have an acid reaction in the system. Ripe fruit, although apparently acid to the taste, has an alkaline reaction in the body, thus interfering with natural digestion.

If You Have An Acid Stomach:
It is extremely important to bear in mind that if refined sugar of any kind, or any flour product is eaten during the same meal with fruits (except bananas, dates, figs or raisins) either together or within an hour or two, the sugars and starches will have a tendency to ferment in the digestive tract, causing an acidulated condition of the stomach.

The Science of Food Combining —
Help Is At Hand
A study of the food chart which is in the back of my book will show how, with a little practice, foods can easily be segregated, and by combining all foods consistently in the manner indicated. a long step in the right direction will have been taken.

This Is One Diet You Can Put Partly Off
Until Tomorrow
I present this matter of food combinations here, at this point, in the hopes of helping you gradually change over from a diet which is cooked and devoid of enzymes, to a way of eating which supplies everything Nature meant us to have for our health and our weight.

I do not advocate as a general rule changing over from customary eating habits in a sudden, complete manner. The reaction from doing so, while generally is more constructive and cleansing to the body, may cause more discomfort (temporarily) than is desired or anticipated.

Unfortunately, we have become a race seeking painkilling remedies for instant relief, disregarding the consequences rather than choosing ways to eradicate the cause of our bodily discomforts by means of the slower, more certain methods.

Which Would You Rather Be Addicted To,
Sleeping Pills or Grapefruit Juice?
For example, insomnia is one of the afflictions daily becoming more pernicious among Americans. Sedatives and sleeping pills of all kinds are increasing in demand. Any drug that induces sleep cannot be anything but habit-forming, advertisements to the contrary, because if the habit is not physical, then it becomes mental. Inability to sleep is sometimes due to malnutrition and toxic conditions in the body reacting on the nerve system, so that the individual loses the power to induce sleep while the toxic conditions exist.

Many sleeping pill drug addicts have found that a large tumbler full of fresh grapefruit juice before going to bed at night, and an enema to clean out the lower intestines, have helped them to the point where they were able to sleep without the use of pills or powders, with little change in their diet. Others have found that a glassful of straight celery juice or lettuce juice worked as efficiently when these juices were properly extracted and taken fresh and raw. A change in the diet is usually effective when concentrated sugars and starches are eliminated.

I am firmly convinced that there is an ever-increasing demand for this knowledge. It is so extremely simple, and yet as old as the hills. More and more people are awakening to the fact that seeking the aid of Nature is to be desired more than blind guessing. After all, except in the case of accident, very little can happen to our body except as a result of what we put into it.

Did You Know Meat Can Give You Bad Breath?

When we eat incompatible mixtures of food, such as meat and potatoes, bread and jam, fruit and sugar, a great deal of fermentation takes place, and the formation of gas is unbelievable.

When, added to the fermentation of such food, we also have the presence of putrefaction of cooked flesh (meat, fish or fowl), the gas is not only increased in volume, but its perfume is anything but esthetic. This accounts for the rank odor which permeates the breath, not only of most meat eating people, but also of most elderly people. When we have corrected our eating habits we will succeed in purifying our breath without the aid of deodorizers.

If You Must, You Must, But I Wouldn't!

When a person actually feels he must have some flesh protein, it has been found that fresh fish with fins and scales have been used with benefit if their cooking has been limited to fifteen minutes of steaming, but not frying it in fat or grease. Sea fish is preferable if fresh, because sea food is the most complete of all foods, and the sea fish contains virtually all the trace elements contained in the oceans.

River and lake fish of the same characteristics, fins and scales, are compatible because lakes and rivers also contain much of the elements washed into them from the mountains, hills and valleys.

Bear in mind, however, that permissible is not the same as total abstinence!

The Man Who Flirted with Death Over a
Piece of Roast Beef and Yorkshire Pudding

The results of the disastrous consequences of the body's inability to handle the deadly combinations of concentrated foods, consumed for years without the slightest notion of the consequences, are very real. Nature has endowed our bodies with the ability to handle much misuse, but there comes a day in which the body's tolerance level has been reached, and we find our bodies breaking down. Our health, which we had taken for granted, has decayed and our bodies are fat and flabby, our muscle tone gone.

There could be no better proof, to my mind, than the case of a man who came under my care, to benefit from my research. He was of British origin, and few meals were complete for him unless they included meat and potatoes and frequently Yorkshire pudding.

He had a stroke a year earlier, which was followed in a comparatively short time by three more. They left him bereft of speech and unable to walk. Orthodox treatments in his home town had left him progressively worse, unable to control his bladder or his bowels.

On his arrival here, I took him to the doctor who at that time cared for my students. As usual, the program was a rigidly strict one: colonic irrigations, quantities of fresh juices daily, raw vegetable and fruits and positively no starchy, sugary or protein foods.

In three months' time, he was able to talk quite coherently and to walk around a little without the aid of even a cane. But his British appetite made his wife's life miserable.

He wanted some meat and potatoes! I told him the chances were that if he did eat such a meal, in three days he would rue the day he was born. Some friends came to visit them the following weekend, and he begged to be able to join them in what he called "a real meal."

"All right," I said, "go ahead if you want to. It's your body, and if you want to suffer the consequences".

They all went to a restaurant famed by publicity for its delicious dinners. There he became a model of decorum by eating only a small piece of meat, a few potatoes, a little bread and a small piece of pie. I met him quite by accident the following Monday, and he was jubilant when he saw me. "See Doc., I told you it wouldn't do me any harm! I feel like a million."

I said, "Fine! I'm glad to hear that. I will remind you of it when I see you on Wednesday."

When I went to their apartment on the following Wednesday, the model of decorum was writhing on his bed, crying like a child. We took him to the doctor who was caring for him, and he was given a colonic irrigation. For nearly a whole hour the gas that poured out of him and the putrid odor of the waste matter washed out of his colon were an object lesson which his wife should never forget as long as she lives.

I reminded them both that I had warned them that, particularity in his condition, flagrantly ignoring his diet would do him no good, and the incompatible combination of the foods he was craving would have exactly the effect we had witnessed.

It is a pitiful and lamentable fact that the vast majority of people simply dig their graves with their teeth, and then eat themselves right into their graves!

When human nature allows the element of appetite to be in control, that person indulges in beverages and foods which are not compatible with natural and physiological laws, and the result is the devastation of the body. The results of this devastation are obvious: pain, ill health, an inclination toward disease, and the outward manifestations of rolls of fatty tissue in the waistline area, with a protruding stomach.

There are so many Americans in this condition, that it has become an almost "normal" state to be in when one reaches their forties, fifties or sixties. It is also true that Americans, are becoming health and weight conscious as never before. But they are pushing their bodies into exercises and the like, without providing the body with the fuel to run on. Exercise is an excellent thing, and it may take off weight, but the nutritional needs of the body must not be neglected, otherwise the body will break down, like a racehorse that has been overworked.

Chapter 17
GETTING STARTED ON NATURAL FOODS
The Correct Definition of Natural Foods

My interpretation of natural foods is that food which is nourishing by virtue of the presence of organic life in it. In this category, I place all raw vegetables and fruits and their fresh, raw, unprocessed juices, and nuts.

Among the vegetables I would also include some of the legumes when they are fresh and young. Dried legumes lack essential organic water, and I have found them to be acid forming in the system. We therefore do not use them. In this class I would include dried peas, beans, soy beans, peanuts, and their many products and by-products.

Whenever possible, we use food that has been grown in organically cultivated ground without the use of industrial chemical fertilizers. While we are not always in a position to choose the quality and the quantity of the vegetables and fruits we need, we can to a great extent overcome this handicap by drinking plenty of fresh raw vegetable juices of as much variety as possible.

Some Favorite Meals From the Walker Household

My purpose in this book has been not only for education as to the kind of foods we should put into our bodies in order to achieve the weight Nature meant for us, but to also provide a practical means to help you get started on Nature's diet plan. I can think of no better way to help you in this endeavor than to share the menus and combinations of foods that I and my wife have as our daily meals.

In the following chapters you will find a most satisfactory recipe section, Fresh Fruit and Raw Vegetable Salads. Also included is a delectable list of various combinations of fresh fruit and vegetable drinks.

As for a typical day's meals in my household, I will give you here an outline of what my own meals consist.

My Favorite Breakfast

For breakfast I have one or two ripe bananas. Ripe bananas are an excellent food, but they must have no green showing, preferably with as much brown in the skin as possible. Cut out any spoiled parts after removing the skin. Slice thinly, or mash with a fork in a soup bowl.

Add 2 or 3 teaspoons of carrot pulp. You can obtain the pulp when you are making carrot juice in your juicer, whether it be a Triturator (pulverizer), or a juicer of the centrifical type. Failing a juicer you can use a simple grater and spread the grated carrot over the bananas.

Next, spread 2 or 3 teaspoons of seedless raisins (soaked overnight in cold or tepid water). Spread 2 or 3 teaspoons over the carrot pulp.

Slice 4-6 black figs (Mission figs are my favorite) over the entire dish. (The figs should be also soaked as you did the raisins.)

I use a nut grinder with which I can grind unsalted almonds almost as fine as flour. If you do not have a nut grinder, you will find it a worthwhile investment, as it has many uses in my recipes. You can obtain one through a health food store.

I spread about 4-5 teaspoons of finely ground almonds over the whole dish, and that is my breakfast.

Should you so desire, you could use some cream, preferably raw, to moisten the food. If so, put it on before spreading the nuts.

A glass of carrot juice or of carrot and spinach juice gives me the best drink I could want to go with a meal.

You will be amazed to find how thoroughly satisfying this breakfast can be. There are many ways in which it can be changed and varied. Using the banana as the base, a sliced or coarsely shredded apple or pear, with raisins and figs as indicated above, with or without the rest of the ingredients, makes a delicious and delightful breakfast.

Personally, I find this the most satisfying breakfast of all. In fact, I doubt if I have changed my menu more than half a dozen times during the past several years. After some practice, I believe that you, too, will find in these suggestions the answer to the kind of breakfast that stays with you, without the discomfort of gas.

What I eat for lunch depends on the circumstances of the day, as I'm sure it does sometimes with you. If I happen to be away from home at lunch time, I take some fruit with me, such as an apple or a pear, or other fruit in season. I also take some celery and a small avocado, if one is available. Otherwise I may occasionally take a small amount of Swiss cheese. This food, together with a pint or two of fresh vegetable juice, gives me all the nourishment I need until dinnertime.

How to Dine Out Without a Fuss

While I am on the subject of meals taken away from home, I must point out that if you have to eat with someone else for lunch or dinner, it is a good idea to be sure to tell your host that you will be bringing along your own "diet" food and that they are not to worry about preparing special foods for you. Actually, it is you who should be worrying about the food they eat! But all the persuasion and campaigning in the world will not be half as effective as the sight of your quietly enjoying your food without a critical word said. Your obvious health and vitality will speak volumes.

Once those friends who do not eat as you do realize that you can be depended upon to "bring your own," they will not feel uncomfortable about inviting you for social occasions. Isn't it strange that we humans have made the consumption of food and drink the center of our social gatherings!

If I am at home for lunch, I eat a small salad consisting of a variety of vegetables. For example,

In a soup dish I may place 2 or 3 tablespoons of carrot pulp. Over this, I spread a mixture of some finely chopped up celery, green onion, cabbage or lettuce, and a little green pepper. Next I add 2 teaspoons of finely shredded beets and about a tablespoon of raw green peas over all. A small piece of raw cauliflower in the middle adds a pleasing artistic touch. You can season to your taste with vegetable salt, which can be bought at your health food store. Apply on each layer.

Try this for a superlative dressing:

$1/3$ cup olive oil

$1/3$ cup lemon juice

3 or 4 medium-sized tomatoes

$1/4$ teaspoon vegetable salt

$1/2$ to 1 teaspoons of honey

Mix these in a liquifer or blender for about 2 minutes. Add about $1/2$ clove of garlic if you are going to use it right away, otherwise put it in a Mason jar and put 2 whole cloves of garlic in to flavor, without breaking them up.

With a glass of vegetable juice, this makes a very satisfying lunch for me, which does not leave me tired and hungry before dinnertime.

You Soon Will Become a Creative Salad Artist

It only takes a short while to make such a salad. If you will remember that all vegetables will mix in a compatible manner, and you have the choice of chopping them fine or coarse, grating them or shredding them, as the case may be, with a little practice you can make a variety of salads with exactly the same vegetables, just prepared differently. In fact, you will be amazed at the ease with which either a simple or an elaborate meal can be prepared. One of the secrets of making a good salad is to mix 2 or 3 vegetables per layer, and use 2 or 3 layers for a salad. This will give you an infinite variety to choose from. Do not use too much, though, of any one vegetable. Just get your vegetables out of your refrigerator and take them as they come, or as they appeal to you, and, with a little practice, you will be able to make a real masterpiece of a salad.

The dinner meals are just as simple to prepare and can be just as plain or elaborate as one desires.

Just Think, No Fighting Over
Who is to Do the Dishes!

You have no idea how much this way of eating simplifies housekeeping! You know what a mess it is to stack up a lot of greasy, dirty dishes, to have to wash and thoroughly sterilize! Then there is the matter of getting the grease cleaned up from the sink. Nature's method of eating does away with nearly all that mess.

Dress Your Salads with Style

Dressings for salads can be made as tasty as they are nourishing. This is true of all the foods that Nature provides. As we are progressing toward a diet which is completely natural, we will find that man-made foods actually taste unnatural, as unnatural as they really are! We will appreciate the wholesome goodness that Nature has to give us.

In the matter of making salad dressings, you will find that they are as creative as salads. You will be using your ingenuity in concocting all kinds of mixtures. Besides the one that I have given you here in this chapter, there are other varieties included in the salad menus.

A Word of Caution About Vinegar

When you do begin to experiment with salad dressings, let me caution you about the use of vinegar. Use only pure apple cider vinegar. In my book, *Fresh Vegetable and Fruit Juices,* I devote a chapter to the matter of vinegars. It recommends the use of apple cider vinegar only, and tells you why you should not use any other!

Desserts: Sweet Mysteries!

Desserts can be as delicious as they can be mystifying when made in a liquifier. For example:

Wow! Is This Good! What Is It?

Put in liquifier:

   1 cup carrot juice
   1 banana cut up in large slices
   2 heaping tablespoons of ground, unsalted almonds
   2 or 3 heaping teaspoons of soaked raisins
   3 or 4 soaked figs
   2-4 tablespoons of cream

Whip this up in the liquifier for about 2 minutes or more. Serve this in a dessert dish, with some whipped cream, if desired.

Chapter 18
PRACTICAL ADVICE AND MORAL SUPPORT

How to Prepare the Various
Vegetables and Fruits

The proportions given in these salads are representative of the average amount for one serving. The vegetables listed below are, of course, raw.

Carrots, Beets, Turnips, Squash, White Radishes, Potatoes, etc.: When a recipe calls for these to be grated, 2 to 4 tablespoons of each is plenty for one ingredient per salad. When shredding is called for use a plain shredder. When diced or sliced, the dimensions should be as small as possible.

Leafy Vegetables: When chopping, use a knife or chopper and cut as finely as possible. They may equally well be passed through a shredder or grinder, and about 1 to 4 tablespoons of each vegetable is ample per portion, according to the number of vegetables in the combination.

Cauliflower: This should be cut into thin slices or it may be chopped finely — about 1 tablespoonful per salad.

Asparagus: Can be chopped finely — use the tips and only as much of the stem as is not too fibrous. Use about 1 tablespoon per helping.

Peppers: Can be grated, chopped or sliced. Use about 1 tablespoon if grated or chopped, or about 4 rings if sliced.

Watercress: Use about 6 to 10 stalks with the leaves on them, per portion.

Avocados: Peel these, then cut into half slices and lay radially on the salad. Usually 6 to 10 slices suffice.

Broccoli: Use same as asparagus.

A Few Tips to a Budding Salad Artist

Almost any combination of raw vegetables and fruits is compatible in salads. If the particular vegetables or fruits mentioned in the following recipes cannot be obtained in your locality, use any others which may be available.

Regulate the amount of each ingredient according to individual taste and capacity. For an average salad, one or two tablespoons of each of the grated or chopped ingredients indicated will suffice. By using fruits and vegetables obtainable locally and using your own initiative and ingenuity, surprisingly delightful salads will result.

Use the following recipes simply as models in the beginning, learning how to prepare and combine the ingredients. Then dispense with the recipes and you will soon be surprised to find how simply you can concoct original and enjoyable salads. When you do begin to try out original ideas in salads it is a good plan, in order to avoid monotony, to use not more than two or three green vegetables, and be sure to include something sweet in the salad.

If any dressing is desired, Health Mayonnaise as described under Salad Dressings, or cottage cheese or honey, or both, will be found to be delicious in that respect.

A Word About Preserving the Non-Preserved Juices

The proper cleaning and sterilizing of the machinery in which juices are made, and all of the utensils and the work area is of paramount importance. Raw vegetable juices are perishable. When first starting on this program it is easy to let that slip our minds, for we are so accustomed to eating and drinking foods with so many chemical preservatives that keep for many weeks in some cases. Because of the freshness in raw, unprocessed juices, every care possible should be taken to make them in a sanitary manner.

When using a home machine, just as in a factory, the juices should never be made in a machine which is not first sterilized with boiling water and then cooled down with cold water. The containers which you will be storing the juices in must also receive this care.

Sometimes juices will spoil in spite of the most meticulous care in sterilizing the equipment. This may be due to the fact that one or more of the vegetables was spoiled, affecting the entire batch. It is, therefore, of extreme importance to clean the vegetables thoroughly and to remove any part that is wilted, discolored or spoiled.

What About Freezing Raw Foods?

While heat in cooking or processing destroys the life element in vegetables, fruits, nuts and other foods, quick freezing does not.

Quick freezing foods that are fresh and tree ripened maintain the life principle in suspension without in any way damaging or destroying the nourishing value of the food.

It is necessary, however, when defrosting such foods, to bear in mind that once their temperature is raised to the point where the life in the atoms composing them become active, they are likely to spoil quicker than in the case of fresh vegetables and fruits from the garden or from the market. The safe temperature to keep such foods after defrosting them is about 34°F. to 38°F., provided they have not been warmed up to room temperature for more than 10 to 15 minutes.

Quick freezing has a tremendous advantage over other methods of keeping foods, as they can be kept frozen for many months without loss or deterioration if the quick freezing temperature is both fast and low enough to thoroughly freeze them. Another desirable feature is the tree or sun ripening of the vegetables and fruits which would make them a perishable product if so marketed without being quick frozen.

Many fruits are sweetened with sugar, and vegetables salted, when quick frozen commercially. It is well to watch for this when buying them, as sugar causes fruits to lose their nourishing value and, as previously said, gives an acid reaction in the body, and salt as an inorganic chemical tends to interfere with the organic processes of digestion.

Now For Some Moral Support:
Be Patient

In the reconstruction and regeneration of the body by natural means, it is very important to bear in mind that natural foods taken in the form of fresh, raw vegetable juices may start a regular housecleaning throughout the entire system. This may be, and sometimes is, accompanied by a period of pains or aches in the regions of the body where this housecleaning is most needed. It may even at times make one feel as if he were actually sick. We should not for one moment feel that the juices are making us ill, especially if they are fresh and are taken on the same day they were made.

On the contrary, we should realize that the cleansing and healing process is well on its way, and the sooner such discomforts are felt after taking plenty of juices, the better — for then we will get over them just so much quicker. The more juices we drink, the faster the recovery.

When in doubt, it is best to consult a doctor whose practice includes an understanding of the therapeutic value of juices. Unless a doctor has used juices consistently, he cannot reasonably be expected to know much about them and their effects. To deprecate or to denounce fresh, raw vegetable juices is to admit a reprehensible lack of knowledge.

We must not expect that a lifetime accumulation of toxins can be squeezed out of our bodies in a miraculous manner.

Don't Let the Uninformed Make You Feel Foolish

It has been claimed by some that carrot juice will turn the skin yellow. It is ignorance of the functions of the body that would make anyone believe such nonsense. It is just as absurd to expect the color pigment of the carrot to come through the skin as to expect the red of the beet or green of the spinach to come through. So be sure to remember that whenever, after drinking juices, yellow or brown appears through the skin, it is an indication that the liver is eliminating stale bile and other waste matter in greater quantities than the eliminative organs can handle, so that some of the elimination takes place through the pores of the skin, which is perfectly normal. If the body is toxic, such also may be the case. Always remember, when we continue to drink vegetable juices, the discoloration disappears.

There are times when, through overwork or excessive exercising and through lack of sleep, even though we feel that our body is in good condition, discoloration may appear. After rest, the discoloration generally vanishes, sooner or later.

In any case, once our body has been regenerated by the continuous use of natural foods and fresh vegetable and fruit juices, and has been cleared of waste and obstructions, we will have such a superabundance of health, energy and vitality that the criticism of uninformed critics will fail to affect us.

Human Nature Vs. Nature

Human nature is often obstinate, stubborn and perverse, refusing to be confused by facts, and is traditionally oblivious to plain common good sense. It seems incomprehensible that supposedly intelligent people can become victimized by claims and statements which misinform and misguide.

Let Nature Write You Out a Prescription

Nature has provided man with all the basic means to enjoy good health and a strong, firm body, devoid of fatty tissue. If we give Nature a chance, we will be rewarded with a state of maximum health, which includes the joy of living with abundant energy, vigor and vitality — and a longer than average span of life!

These basic means which Nature provides are few, but they are simple and effective. First, Nature's means are physically represented in our natural foods as Nature intended them to be eaten. Second, if we have let our bodies become fat and unhealthy, Nature provides a means to begin rebuilding our bodies through the understanding of the importance of keeping the body's eliminative system clean and free of substances which, if allowed to remain in the colon for any length of time, will result in putrefaction and fermentation.

Third, Nature's means to a fulfilling life also includes a healthy, positive outlook on life. Food and the state of the mind work hand in hand. The very best of food becomes a poison in the system when negative emotions are present during eating. When one is tired, angry, worried, fearful, jealous, or in any other such state of consciousness, one should refrain from eating or drinking anything, until one can become rested and calm. To put food in the system at such negative times causes unpredictable reactions. The food does not digest properly, and the result is toxemia.

On the other hand, when a happy, cheerful, sunny atmosphere prevails during a meal, even little things that might otherwise annoy one are readily overlooked and discounted, so that the meal is a pleasant affair and the digestion responds in kind. The entire alimentary tract becomes buoyant and responsive, while at the same time the eliminative organs are ready to take care of the waste from the body. The result is the assimilation of food in the best manner.

When we adapt a positive outlook on life, we are in control of life. This does not mean that we get everything we want. That, as a matter of fact, might be the worst thing that could happen to us. It does mean that we have learned to balance what we want, against what comes our way. It means that we have learned to put up with people and conditions which surround us, realizing that nothing is permanent except change!

Nature Doesn't Neglect the Soul

Happiness, peace and security are sought after by everybody. These conditions cannot be found in external circumstances. They cannot be found outside of ourselves. Until we have found and developed them from within our hearts and minds, we will continue to seek in vain.

Once we have discovered how simple it is to find these in our own consciousness, we get an entirely new perspective on life. We will have attained a state of sublime self-reliance and self-sufficiency which no one can take away from us. Otherwise, we can lose all the weight we want, but the change will only be outward. What good is a healthy body and an ideal weight if there is no change from within? Inside you will still be that overweight person who had one health problem after another.

If you learn to be in control of your life, you will sparkle with an inner radiance reflected in your eyes and in your personality. You will be a supreme example of the work that you, through Nature's plan, strived to achieve - and succeeded!

FRESH FRUIT AND VEGETABLE SALAD RECIPES

NOTE: Recipes 1-50 are single serving.

No. 1

Carrots, 2 tablespoons	— finely grated
Lettuce, 2 tablespoons	— finely chopped
Tomato, ½ medium-sized	— divided into small segments
Celery, 2 tablespoons	— finely chopped
Persimmon, ⅔ medium-sized	— peeled and divided into segments
Raisins, 2 tablespoons	— Thompson seedless preferably
Red cabbage, 2 tablespoons	— finely chopped
Banana, ½ large one	— diced
Dates, 2 large or 3 small	— cut into small segments
Radishes, 5 small	— finely sliced
Apple, 1 large	— shredded (preferably Delicious)
Avocado, ½ medium-sized	— peeled and sliced lengthwise

For garnish — 1 date, chopped walnuts, maraschino cherry, watercress.

Arrange each in layer beginning with carrots, one on top of the other up to and including the banana. Place radishes around the side of dish, grated apple in the center, avocado slices around sides, one date quartered and placed cross-like in the center, nuts sprinkled over the top and maraschino cherry in center. Garnish around edge of salad with watercress.

No. 2

Celery, 2 tablespoons	— finely chopped
Carrot, 2 tablespoons	— finely grated
Lettuce, 2 tablespoons	
Onion, 1 tablespoon	— finely chopped and mixed together
Tomato, ½ medium-sized	
Red cabbage, 2 tablespoons	— finely chopped
Banana squash, 1 tablespoon	— finely grated
Apple, 1 Delicious, shredded	
Fig, 1 large, cut in segments	Mix all together.
Honey, 2 teaspoons	
Walnuts, 2 tablespoons, chopped	
Avocado, ½ medium-sized	— peeled and sliced lengthwise
Radishes, 5 small	— use whole
Olives, stuffed	
Parsley	

Arrange in several layers as follows — celery, then carrot, the mixture of lettuce, onion, tomato and red cabbage. In the center place the banana squash, apple, figs, honey and walnuts. Place avocado slices and radishes around sides, stuffed olives in center and garnish with parsley.

No. 3

Asparagus (raw), 1 or 2 stalks, fresh and crisp
String beans (raw), 6 fresh and crisp — chopped finely
Lettuce, ¼ head, fresh and crisp — coarsely chopped
Parsley, 2 tablespoons — finely minced
Carrot, 1 small — finely grated
Cottage cheese, Farmer's style preferably, 2 ounces
Peach, ½ large fresh
Avocado, ½ medium-sized — peeled and cut lengthwise
Lettuce leaves
Pecan and walnut halves, 4 or 5

Mix all of above together in a bowl, except the peach, avocado, some of the nut meats and a little of the cottage cheese. Arrange crisp leaves of lettuce on dinner plate and place this mixture on plate in the form of a mound. Cover the mound with thin slices of peach and garnish with thin slices of the avocado. Place the remaining cottage cheese in the center and sprinkle with finely chopped nut meats.

No. 4

Lettuce, ¼ head crisp and fresh — coarsely chopped
Celery, 2 or 3 stalks — finely chopped
Cucumber, ½ large (do not peel) — finely grated
Parsley, 1 tablespoon — finely minced
Onions, green, 3 or 4 small — finely chopped
Asparagus (raw), 2 or 3 stalks, fresh and crisp — finely chopped
Cauliflower, 2 teaspoons — finely grated
Peas, fresh tender green, 1 or 2 tablespoons — use whole
Avocado, ½ medium-sized
Lettuce leaves

Arrange crisp leaves of lettuce on dinner plate and place the above vegetables in layers, each in the order given, sprinkling the green peas over the top and garnishing with the strips of avocado. (If the cucumber is grated, including the peeling, this makes the peeling very fine and easy to masticate and also brings out the juice of the cucumber giving moisture and flavor to the salad.)

No. 5

Lettuce, ¼ head crisp, fresh
Celery, 1 or 2 stalks — chopped fine
Irish potato, (raw with skin on) ½ small — diced very small
Carrot, 1 medium-sized — finely grated
Onion, Sweet Spanish, ½ large size — finely chopped
Green pepper, 1 teaspoon — finely chopped
Tomatoes, 2 small or 1 large ripe — peeled and cut in thin slices
Cottage cheese, preferably Farmer Style, 2 ounces
Avocado, ½ medium-sized — peeled, cut lengthwise
Lettuce leaves or endive

Arrange all the chopped and grated vegetables in mound on crisp leaves of lettuce or endive, cover with slices of tomato, garnish with strips of avocado and top with mound of cottage cheese sprinkled with paprika.

No. 6

Lettuce, ½ head solid, crisp	— chopped
Avocado, ½ large	— peeled and sliced lengthwise
Pineapple, 4 slices (preferably fresh or canned unsweetened)	
Cottage Cheese, 3 ounces (preferably Farmer Style)	
Parsley, 1 tablespoon	— finely minced
Red pepper, sweet, few strips	
Endive or lettuce leaves	

Arrange chopped lettuce on bed of endive or lettuce leaves and cover with layer of cottage cheese. Arrange strips of avocado across the center of the dish and place strips of pineapple on either side. Sprinkle very finely chopped parsley over all this and garnish with thin strips of sweet red pepper. (The avocado may be sliced with a wire egg slicer.)

No. 7

Lettuce, ½ head, solid, crisp	— chopped fine
Carrots, 1 or 2 large crisp	— finely grated
Raisins, seedless, ¼ cup	
Cottage Cheese, 3 ounces	
Honey	

Arrange chopped lettuce on plate or dish, cover with grated carrot and one-half of raisins mixed together. Sprinkle with 1 teaspoon or more of honey, cover with cottage cheese and garnish with the balance of the raisins.

No. 8

Cabbage, ½ cup, fresh crisp	— finely chopped
Celery, ½ cup	— diced
Spinach, 3 or 4 leaves	— finely chopped
Carrot, 1 large	— finely grated
Honey, 1 tablespoon	
Cottage Cheese, 2 or 3 ounces	
Apples, 1 large grated or grated unsweetened pineapple	
Parsley, 1 tablespoon	— finely minced
Red sweet pepper, 1 large or radish rings for garnish.	

Arrange layers of cabbage, celery and spinach on dinner plate. Cover this with the grated carrots and sprinkle as evenly as possible with 1 tablespoonful of honey, cover with cottage cheese and top with grated apple or pineapple. Garnish with sprigs of parsley and strips of red sweet pepper or radish rings.

No. 9

String beans (raw and fresh), 6 or 7	— grated fine
Asparagus, (raw and fresh), 4 or 5 stalks	— chopped fine
Cucumbers, ½ large (including skin)	— grated fine
Green pepper, 1 teaspoon	— grated
Celery, 2 or 3 stalks, crisp	— grated or finely chopped
Carrots, 1 or 2 large crisp	— finely grated
Pecan meats, ¼ cup	— finely chopped
Grapes, Thompson Seedless, ½ cup	— cut in halves or quarters
Peach, 1 large fresh ripe	— slice thinly lengthwise

Mix all the above ingredients together in bowl, except the peach, nuts and a few grapes. Arrange mixture on crisp lettuce leaves, cover with sliced peaches and garnish with nuts and grapes cut in halves. Honey may be added if desired.

No. 10

Lettuce, ¼ head	— chopped
Asparagus (raw fresh), 2 or 3 stalks	— finely chopped
Green onions, 4 or 5 or	
Sweet Spanish onion, ½ large	— finely chopped
Green pepper, 1 tablespoon	— finely chopped
Celery, 2 or 3 stalks, crisp	— finely chopped
Tomatoes, 2 medium-sized, firm ripe	— peeled and sliced
Cottage cheese, 2 ounces	

Mix these all together except the tomatoes and a little of the cottage cheese. Arrange in mound on crisp leaves of lettuce and cover with thin slices of tomato. Top with cottage cheese and a dash of paprika.

No. 11

Irish potato (raw with skin), ½ medium sized	— finely grated
Carrots, 1 small	— finely grated
Celery, 2 or 3 stalks, crisp	— finely chopped
Parsley, 1 tablespoon	— finely minced
Green pepper, 1 teaspoon	— finely grated
Apples, 1 large juicy	— grated
Beets, 2 medium-sized young	— grated finely
Nuts, ¼ cupful (pecans or walnuts)	— finely chopped

Mix these all together except the apples and beets and a few of the nuts. Arrange this mixture on crisp leaves of lettuce, cover with layer of grated apple and top with layer of grated beets sprinkled with the chopped nuts.

No. 12

Red cabbage, ½ cup	— finely chopped
Asparagus, 3 or 4 stalks	— finely cut
Green onions, 3 or 4	— finely chopped
Celery, 3 or 4 stalks, fresh crisp	— grated or finely chopped
String beans (raw fresh), 4 or 5	— grated
Tomatoes, 2 large, firm ripe	— peeled, one sliced, one diced
Green pepper, 1 teaspoon	— finely grated
Cottage cheese, 2 ounces	
Marjoram (herb)	
Cucumber, ½ medium sized	— slice thinly
Paprika	

Mix cabbage, asparagus, onions, celery, string beans, the diced tomato, green pepper and most of the cottage cheese, together in a bowl. Sprinkle lightly with Marjoram (one of the herbs which can be bought at grocery stores in powdered form). Arrange in a mound on plate garnished with lettuce leaves or endive and cover with the remaining sliced tomato and top with remaining cottage cheese. Arrange the cucumber slices around outer edge of salad. Add a dash of paprika to the cottage cheese and cucumber slices.

No. 13

Red cabbage, 1 tablespoon	— finely chopped
Lettuce, ¼ head crisp	— finely chopped
Celery, 2 tablespoons	— finely cut
Parsley, 1 tablespoon	— finely minced
Green pepper, ¼ teaspoon	— finely grated
Beets, 1 or 2 tablespoons young tender	— finely grated
Avocado, ½ large	— peeled and cut lengthwise
Cottage cheese, 1 tablespoon (Farmer's style)	— made into two balls
Paprika	
Ripe olives	

Celery stuffed with avocado paste to which has been added ground almonds.

Mix cabbage, lettuce, celery, parsley and green pepper together and form in mound. Place in center of plate garnished with crisp lettuce leaves or endive, top with grated beet and surround with slices of avocado, arranging the two cottage cheese balls, sprinkled with paprika, on either side of the mound. Serve with ripe olives, and crisp celery stuffed with avocado paste and almonds (made by mashing ripe avocado and whipping to smooth creamy consistency, then mixing in finely chopped or ground almonds).

No. 14

Lettuce, ½ head, crisp fresh	— finely chopped
Spinach, 6 or 8 leaves	— finely chopped
Parsley, 1 tablespoon	— finely minced
Green onions, 6 or 8	— finely chopped
Watercress	
Cucumber, ½ large, fresh, crisp and unpeeled	

Garnish plates with lettuce leaves or endive. Mix spinach, parsley, onions and watercress together and sprinkle over this. Cover with sliced cucumbers and a dash of paprika.

No.15

Green onions, 3 or 4	— finely chopped
Romaine lettuce, 3 or 4 crisp leaves	— finely chopped
Parsley, 1 tablespoon	— finely minced
Radishes, 3 or 4, fresh crisp	— finely cut
Celery, 3 or 4 stalks	— finely chopped
Asparagus, 3 or 4 stalks (raw)	— finely cut
Peas, fresh tender green (raw), ¼ cup	— whole
Cucumber, ½ medium-sized incl. peel	— grated
Tomatoes, 1 medium-sized, firm red	— peeled and cut in wedges

Mix these all together, except the tomatoes, and arrange in mound on leaves of lettuce or endive. Surround with wedges of tomato. Swiss cheese is delicious served with this.

No. 16

Lettuce, ½ small, firm crisp head	— finely chopped
Celery, 2 or 3 stalks	— finely chopped
Parsley, 2 tablespoons	— finely chopped
Parsley, 2 tablespoons	— finely minced
Tomatoes, 2 medium-sized, firm ripe	— peeled and sliced
Avocado, ½ large ripe	— peeled and sliced lengthwise

Garnish plate with endive and cover this with the chopped lettuce, celery and parsley. Garnish with sliced tomatoes and avocado arranged alternately.

No. 17

Lettuce, ¼ head, crisp	— finely chopped
String beans, (raw) fresh green, 4 or 5	— finely chopped
Cucumber, ½ large with skin	— grated
Watercress, 3 or 4 sprigs	— finely minced
Green pepper, 1 teaspoon	— finely grated
Tomatoes, 1 large, ripe firm	— peeled and sliced
Avocado, ½ medium-sized	— peeled and sliced lengthwise
Cottage cheese, 2 ounces	

Mix all the chopped and grated vegetables together and arrange in mound on crisp lettuce. Cover with sliced tomatoes and arrange slices of avocado around edge. Top with the cottage cheese.

No. 18

Tomatoes, 1 very large, smooth, red, firm	— cut off the top, scoop out the center and scallop the top edge
Celery, 3 or 4 stalks, crisp	— finely chopped
Green onions, 3 or 4	— finely chopped
Cucumber, ½ medium-sized, with peel	— grated
Cottage cheese, 2 ounces	
Ripe olives, 4 large	
Green pepper, sweet	

After scalloping edge of tomato, cut down through the scallops to form flower-like petals and spread open on plate garnished with endive. Mix the scooped out portion of the tomato, chopped celery, green onions and enough cottage cheese to hold the mixture together. Fill the center of the tomato with this mixture. Top with the balance of the cottage cheese and garnish with very thin strips of sweet green pepper and ripe olives.

No. 19

Celery, 3 or 4 stalks, crisp	— finely minced
Avocado, ½ large, ripe	
Apples, 1 very large or 2 small	— peeled, cored and sliced in rings less than ¼ inch thick, dip in lemon juice to prevent browning.
Parsley, 1 tablespoon	— finely chopped

Arrange the chopped celery on beds of endive or crisp lettuce leaves. Peel the avocado and cut in thin rings around the pit. Place one avocado ring on top of each apple ring. Arrange these decoratively over the bed of chopped celery and sprinkle with minced parsley. Strips of Swiss cheese may be served with this.

No. 20

Cabbage, 1 cup, crisp	— finely chopped
Celery, 2 or 3 stalks	— finely chopped
Ripe olives, 5 or 6, large	
Radishes, red, small, crisp 4 or 5	— cut into small pieces
Sour cream	

Mix these all together, saving a few radishes for garnishing. Mix sour cream into the vegetables, using enough to suit the individual's taste. If it tastes flat add a little vegetable salt. Serve on romaine lettuce bed, garnishing top with very thin slices of radishes.

No. 21

Lettuce, ¼ head, crisp	— chopped
Celery, 3 or 4 stalks	— finely chopped
Persimmons, 1 large or 2 small, very ripe	— peeled and cut in sections
Cottage cheese, 2 or 3 ounces	
Date, ½ large for garnish	

Arrange lettuce and celery on endive, cover with sections of persimmon and top with the cottage cheese with half of date in center.

No. 22

Lettuce, ½ small, crisp head	— finely chopped
Celery, 2 stalks	— finely chopped
Prunes, fresh or dried*, ½ cup	— cut from seeds into small pieces
Apples, 1 large, ripe juicy	— finely grated
Cream, ½ cup, sweet whipped. (preferably raw)	— sweeten with honey
Walnuts	

Mix together the celery, lettuce, prunes and apples and add enough whipped cream, sweetened with honey, to make the right consistency. Serve on crisp beds of lettuce topped with the balance of the whipped cream and finely cut walnut meats.

*If dried prunes are used, soak them in tepid water overnight or until soft. Do not cook.

No. 23

Tomatoes, 1 or 2 large, firm ripe	— peeled and cut in wedge-like sections
Avocado, ½ large or 1 small, ripe	— peeled and cut lengthwise
Cottage cheese, 2 or 3 ounces	
Endive	

Arrange endive on dinner plate and alternate tomato sections with slices of avocado around outer edge. Mould cottage cheese in center with a dash of paprika.

No. 24

Pineapple, ½ cup, unsweetened tidbits	
Pear, ½ medium-sized	— grated
Apple, 1 small (Delicious preferable)	— grated
Cabbage, ½ cup, crisp	— finely chopped
Pecans	
Cream, ½ cup, sweet whipped, (preferably raw)	— sweetened with honey

Mix pineapple, pear, apple and cabbage lightly with two forks. Add about half of the whipped cream. Arrange on bed of crisp lettuce and garnish with balance of the whipped cream and pecans.

No. 25

Cabbage, ½ cup, crisp	— finely chopped
Parsley, 1 tablespoon	— finely minced
Celery, 2 stalks, crisp	— finely chopped
Carrots, 1 large	— finely chopped
Honey, 1 tablespoon	
Cottage cheese, 2 ounces	
Apples, 1 small or medium-sized (Delicious)	— grated
Avocado, ½ small	— peeled and cut lengthwise

Arrange above in order given on bed of lettuce using avocado around edge for garnish, a sprig of parsley or watercress may be placed in center.

No. 26

Turnips, 1 medium-sized, sweet young white	— grated
Red cabbage, ½ cup, crisp	— finely chopped
Celery, 1 or 2 stalks, crisp	— finely chopped
Parsley, 1 tablespoon	— finely minced
Romaine lettuce, ½ small head	— finely chopped
Avocado, ½ medium-sized	— peeled and cut lengthwise

Mix these all together with a little Health Mayonnaise, tossing lightly with two forks, and serve on boats made of Romaine lettuce leaves, garnished with sliced avocado, sprinkled with paprika.

No. 27

No. 1

Cabbage, ½ cup, crisp	— finely chopped
Green pepper, 1 teaspoon	— finely chopped
Celery, 1 or 2 stalks, crisp	— finely chopped
Sour cream dressing	

No. 2

Celery, 4 or 5 stalks, crisp	— finely chopped
Carrot, 1 small	— finely grated
Health Mayonnaise	

No. 3

Celery, 1 or 2 stalks, crisp	— finely chopped
Beet, 1 medium-sized, young tender	— finely grated
Lettuce, ½ head, small crisp	— finely chopped

For garnish: 3 or 4 small red radishes, ¼ avocado and green pepper.

Mix the three above combinations separately in the order in which the ingredients are listed, using the amount of dressing desired in each, and place in moulds. Arrange endive on a large dinner plate and unmould these three combinations in center, leaving at least 1 inch space between them, so they will not be jumbled together. Garnish No. 1 with thin slices of crisp red radishes; No. 2 with spears of avocado and No. 3 with thin strips of green pepper and one stuffed olive. Serve with stuffed olives, Swiss cheese and celery hearts.

No. 28

Cabbage, ⅓ cup, crisp	— finely chopped
Celery, 3 or 4 stalks	— finely chopped
Lettuce, ¼ small crisp head	— finely chopped
Carrot, 1 medium-sized	— finely grated
Green pepper, 1 teaspoon	— finely chopped
Sour cream dressing	
Marjoram, a dash	
Cottage cheese, 2 ounces	

For garnish: ¼ avocado cut in strips, and sweet red pepper strips.

Mix vegetables together with sour cream to suit taste, tossing lightly with two forks. Arrange this mixture in a mound in the center of crisp lettuce or endive with a dash of Marjoram over all. Top with cottage cheese and garnish with avocado and sweet red pepper strips. Serve with celery stuffed with cream cheese and chopped pecans.

No. 29

Bananas, 1 or 2 very ripe	— diced
Lettuce, ¼ small, crisp head	— finely chopped
Celery, 2 or 3 stalks, crisp	— finely chopped
Raisins, seedless, 1 tablespoon	
Pear, ½ ripe firm	— diced
Cream, sweet whipped, ½ cup (preferably raw)	— sweetened with honey
Nuts (pecans or walnuts) 2 tablespoons	— finely chopped

Mix all ingredients with part of the whipped cream and some of the nuts, and arrange in mound on crisp lettuce or endive. Top with balance of whipped cream and nuts.

No. 30

Apples, 1 or 2 ripe juicy Jonathans	— grated finely
Spinach, 5 or 6 leaves, crisp fresh	— finely chopped
Celery, 3 or 4 stalks	— finely chopped
Red cabbage, 1/3 cup	— finely chopped
Parsley, 1 tablespoon	— finely minced

Mix half of grated apple with chopped vegetables, except parsley. Arrange in center of bed of crisp lettuce and cover with remaining apple and minced parsley. With this may be served thin slices of Swiss cheese.

No. 31

Grapefruit, 1 large ripe sweet	— peel and remove membrane from sections
Avocado, ½ large ripe but firm	— peel and cut lengthwise
Lettuce, ½ small solid crisp head	— finely chopped
Celery, 3 or 4 stalks	— finely chopped
Cottage cheese, 2 or 3 ounces	
Pecans, 1 tablespoon	— finely chopped, leaving one whole for garnish

Garnish dinner plate with crisp lettuce or endive and make a graceful wheel around outer edge, using grapefruit sections and thin slices of avocado alternately. Mix together the chopped lettuce and celery, half of the cottage cheese and all but the one pecan. Arrange this in center of plate and top with balance of the cottage cheese and the pecan. Add a dash of paprika.

No. 32

Spinach, ½ large fresh bunch	— very finely chopped
Avocado, ½ large ripe	— peeled and mashed until fluffy
Celery, 2 or 3 stalks	— finely chopped
Onion, sweet Spanish, ¼ medium-sized	— finely chopped
Tomatoes, 2 medium-sizedripe firm red	— scoop out centers
Ripe olives and green sweet pepper for garnish	

Mix together the spinach, avocado, celery and onion and fill tomato cups. Place on dinner plate on bed of endive and garnish top with thin strips of green sweet pepper and place ripe olive in center of each stuffed tomato. This may be served with celery hearts, ripe olives and strips of Swiss cheese.

No. 33

Spinach, ½ large bunch	— very finely chopped
Apples, 1 or 2 small juicy	— finely grated
Persimmons, 1 large or 2 small, very ripe	— peeled and cut in sections
Celery, 2 or 3 stalks	— finely chopped
Cottage cheese, 1 or 2 tablespoons	
Avocado, ½ small	— peeled and cut lengthwise

Mix spinach, apples, persimmons and celery together and serve on bed of lettuce topped with cottage cheese and garnished with strips of avocado and a dash of paprika.

No. 34

Lettuce, ½ small crisp solid head	— finely chopped
Cabbage, ¼ cup, crisp	— finely chopped
Irish potato (raw), ¼ medium-sized	— finely grated
Almonds, ¼ cup	— grated or ground
Green pepper, sweet, 1 teaspoon	— finely chopped
Cottage cheese, 1 or 2 ounces	
Pecan halves, 6 or 8	
Avocado, ½ small	— peeled and cut lengthwise
Dash of Marjoram	

Mix together the lettuce, cabbage, potato, green pepper, Marjoram and almonds and arrange on bed of crisp lettuce or endive. Cover outer edge of mound with slices of avocado and pecan halves. Top with cottage cheese and dash of paprika.

No. 35

Carrots, 1 medium-sized	— finely grated
Spinach, ½ bunch, fresh crisp	— finely chopped
Lettuce, ¼ head, firm crisp	— finely chopped
Parsley, 1 tablespoon	— finely minced
Cottage cheese, 2 or 3 ounces	
Cream	
Honey, 1 teaspoon	
Dates, 4 or 5	— finely chopped
Apple, 1 large Delicious	— grated
Avocado, ¼ medium-sized	— peeled and cut lengthwise

Mix together in a bowl the carrots, spinach, lettuce and parsley and to this add about 1 tablespoon of cottage cheese to which enough cream has been added to make it the consistency of salad dressing. Place this mixture on bed of crisp lettuce on dinner plate, sprinkle with honey and cover with layer of chopped dates. Add layer of grated apple and top with balance of cottage cheese and strips of avocado with a dash of paprika.

No. 36

Cabbage, ⅓ cup, crisp	— finely chopped
Celery, 3 or 4 stalks, fresh crisp	— finely chopped
Parsley, 1 tablespoon	— finely minced
Honey, 1 teaspoon	
Apple, 1 large Delicious	— grated
Banana, ½ large ripe	— thinly sliced
Persimmons, 1 medium or 2 small, ripe	— peel and cut lenghtwise
Cottage cheese, 1 or 2 ounces	

Ganish dinner plate with endive and arrange the above in layers in the order given except persimmons and cottage cheese. Arrange sections of persimmons and around outer edge of layers and top with cottage cheese, with sprig of parsley of watercress in center.

No. 37

Spinach, ½ bunch, fresh crisp	— finely chopped
Lettuce, ¼ small crisp head	— finely chopped
Celery, 2 or 3 stalks	— finely chopped
Avocado, ⅓ large	— peel, mash and beat until light and fluffy
Carrots, 1 large	— finely grated
Honey, 1 teaspoon	
Cottage cheese, 2 or 3 ounces	
Apple, 1 medium sized juicy	— grated
Parsley, 1 tablespoon	— chopped

Mix together the spinach, lettuce, celery and mashed avocado and arrange a layer of this on dinner plate garnished with crisp leaves of lettuce or endive. Cover this with layer of grated carrots, sprinkle with honey and add layer of cottage cheese, then grated apple, and garnish with chopped parsley.

No. 38

Cabbage, ⅓ cup, crisp	— finely chopped
Dates, 5 or 6	— finely chopped
Parsley, 1 tablespoon	— finely minced
Lettuce, ¼ head solid crisp	— finely chopped
Watercress, several sprigs	— finely minced
Honey, 1 teaspoon	
Apple, 1 large or medium-sized Delicious	— grated
Cottage cheese, 2 or 3 ounces	
Avocado, ¼ large	— peeled and cut lengthwise
Paprika, a dash	

Garnish dinner plate with endive or crisp leaves of lettuce and cover with layer of cabbage, then dates and parsley, lettuce and watercress and sprinkle with honey. Cover this with layer of apple, then cottage cheese. Arrange thin slices of avocado around outer edge of mound, place sprig of parsley in center. Add a dash of paprika.

No. 39

Lettuce, ¼ head, solid crisp	— finely chopped
Celery, 2 or 3 stalks	— finely chopped
Carrot, 1 medium-sized	— grated
Figs, *Black Mission, 3 or 4	— finely cut
Watercress, several sprigs	— finely chopped
Honey, 1 teaspoon	
Cottage cheese, 2 or 3 ounces	
Apple, 1 large or medium-sized, juicy	— finely grated

Arrange Romaine lettuce on dinner plate and add layers of lettuce, celery, carrots, figs and watercress. Sprinkle with honey and cover with cottage cheese, topping with grated apple and sprig of watercress.

*If dried figs are used, soak until soft in tepid water; do not cook.

No. 40

Celery, 3 or 4 stalks	— finely chopped
Lettuce, ¼ small crisp head	— finely chopped
Parsley, 1 tablespoonful	— finely minced .
Honey, 1 teaspoon	
Beets, 2 small or 1 medium, fresh tender	— finely grated
Apple, 1 large, Delicious	— grated
Cottage cheese, 2 or 3 ounces	
Paprika, a dash	

Arrange layer of celery, lettuce and parsley on bed of crisp endive and sprinkle with honey. Cover with layer of grated beets, then apple and top with cottage cheese and a dash of paprika with a sprig of parsley in center.

No. 41

Winter pears, 2 large, juicy	— cut in cubes
Lettuce, ½ head, crisp firm	— cut in medium sized chunks
Dates, 5 or 6	— finely cut
Cream, sweet whipped, ½ cup (preferably raw)	— sweetened with honey
Romaine lettuce	

Mix enough of whipped cream with pears, lettuce and dates to suit the individual taste and serve in boats made of Romaine lettuce. Top with the balance of whipped cream and one-half date.

No. 42

Carrots, 2 tablespoons	— finely grated
Spinach, 2 tablespoons	— finely chopped
Banana, ½ medium-sized ripe	— diced
Raisins, 2 tablespoons	
Red cabbage, 2 tablespoons	— finely chopped
Lettuce, 2 tablespoons, crisp fresh	— finely chopped
Green pepper, 2 tablespoons	— finely chopped
Persimmon, ½ large	— peeled and divided in segments
Apple, 1 medium-sized Delicious	— grated
Avocado, ⅓ medium-sized, ripe	— peeled and cut lengthwise
Parsley, several sprigs	
Almonds, raw, 8 or 10	— whole or chopped

Place on crisp lettuce leaves a layer of grated carrot, then spinach, and spread each of the other ingredients one on top of the other in the order mentioned. The persimmon segments may be arranged around the center of mixture and the slices of avocado radially around this, using parsley and whole or chopped almonds for garnish.

No. 43

Cabbage, 2 tablespoons	— finely chopped
Spinach, 2 tablespoons	— finely chopped
Celery, 2 tablespoons	— finely chopped
Broccoli, 1 tablespoon	— finely chopped
Peas, raw, fresh, tender and green, 2 tablespoons	
Cottage cheese, 2 ounces	
Honey	
Apple, 1 medium-sized Delicious	— finely grated
Green pepper, 1 ring	
Radish, 1 medium or large red	

Arrange above in a large soup dish, layer by layer in order given. Sprinkle the cottage cheese with honey before adding the grated apple. Save out two teaspoons of cottage cheese for garnish. Lay green pepper ring in center of apple layer, place cottage cheese in center and top with the radish.

No. 44

Lettuce, 2 tablespoons	— finely chopped
Celery, 2 tablespoons	— finely chopped
Spinach, 2 tablespoons	— finely chopped
Green pepper, 1 tablespoon	— finely chopped
Peas, raw fresh, tender and green, 2 tablespoons	
Cottage cheese, 2 ounces	
Honey	
Apple, 1 medium-sized Delicious	— finely grated
Cauliflower, ¼ head	— divided into small cauliflowerettes
Radishes, red, 3 made into roses*	
Avocado, ½ medium-sized	

*this is done by thoroughly cleaning radishes, cut off top, take one slice from tail end and with paring knife gently peel the red skin back like petals from the tail end.

Arrange in large soup dish by layers the lettuce, celery, spinach, green pepper and peas. Dot with cottage cheese and sprinkle with honey. Save about one teaspoon of cottage cheese for garnish. Add the apple, finely grated. Place the cauliflower in center. Divide the cottage cheese into three dabs in equal distances around cauliflower and place a radish rose in center of each dab. Arrange thick slices of avocado around outer edge.

No. 45

Cabbage, 2 tablespoons	— finely chopped
Lettuce, 2 tablespoons	— finely chopped
Celery, 2 tablespoons	— finely chopped
Broccoli, 1 tablespoon	— finely chopped
Spinach, 1 tablespoon	— finely chopped
Green pepper, 1 ring	
Cottage cheese, 2 ounces	
Honey	
Apple, 1 medium-sized, sweet and ripe	— finely grated
Radish, red, 1 rose (see salad No. 44)	

Arrange finely chopped vegetables in layers on plate or in large soup dish, top with half the cottage cheese, sprinkle with honey, cover with the apple, finely grated. Arrange balance of cottage cheese in mound in center and on top of this place green pepper ring with the radish rose in center.

106

No. 46

Beet, 2 tablespoons, red and sweet, raw	— very finely grated
Celery, 2 tablespoons	— diced
Cabbage, 2 tablespoons	— finely chopped
Apple, 1 medium, sweet	— diced
Whipped cream, 2 tablespoons	
Walnuts, 2 tablespoons	— finely cut or sliced
Honey	

Mix together the grated beet, celery, cabbage, apple and half the whipped cream (which has been sweetened to taste with honey). Arrange in soup dish and top with remaining whipped cream and sprinkle the chopped or sliced walnuts over it all.

No. 47

Cabbage, 2 tablespoons	— finely chopped
Celery, 2 tablespoons	— finely chopped
Broccoli, 1 tablespoon	— finely chopped
Cauliflower, 1 tablespoon	— finely chopped
Spinach, 1 tablespoon	— finely chopped
Cottage cheese, 2 ounces	
Apple, 1 medium-sized, sweet	— finely grated
Green pepper, 1 ring	
Red pepper, sweet, 2 rings	
Honey	

Arrange the chopped vegetables in soup dish in layers in order given above. Top with half of cottage cheese, sprinkle with honey, add layer of grated apple and place remaining cottage cheese in center, topped with green pepper ring. Cut the two red pepper rings in half, arrange three of the halves around edge of salad and dice the fourth half on top of cottage cheese, inside green pepper ring.

No. 48

Cabbage, 2 tablespoons	— finely chopped
Celery, 2 tablespoons	— finely chopped
Cauliflower, 1 tablespoon	— finely chopped
Carrot, 1 tablespoon	— finely grated
Broccoli, 1 tablespoon	— finely chopped
Spinach, 1 tablespoon	— finely chopped
Cottage cheese, 2 ounces	
Honey	
Apple, 1 medium-sized sweet	— grated
Green pepper, 2 rings	
Radishes, 3 red	
Olive, 1 ripe	

Arrange the chopped and grated vegetables in layers in soup dish in order given. Top with half the cottage cheese, sprinkle with honey, cover with layer of finely grated apple. Arrange green pepper rings around outer edge of salad and place a radish in center of each. Put remaining cottage cheese in middle of salad and top with the ripe olive.

Cabbage, 2 tablespoons	— finely chopped
Spinach, 2 tablespoons	— finely chopped
Celery, 2 tablespoons	— finely chopped
Summer squash, 1 medium-sized green scalloped, raw	— diced
Cottage cheese, 2 ounces	
Tomatoes, 2 medium-sized or 1 large	— sliced
Green pepper, 2 rings	

The chopped vegetables can be arranged in layers, add the diced summer squash, half the cottage cheese and top with the sliced tomatoes. Garnish with the balance of cottage cheese and green pepper rings.

No. 50

Cabbage, 2 tablespoons	— finely chopped
Spinach, New Zealand (or regular) 1 tablespoon	— finely chopped
Celery, 2 tablespoons	— finely chopped
Cottage cheese, 2 ounces	
Tomatoes, 2 medium-sized or 1 large firm, ripe	— sliced
Green pepper, 1 ring	
Radish, 1 red	
Summer squash, Zucchini, 2 tablespoons, raw	— diced
Cucumber, ½ medium-sized	— diced
Onion, Sweet Spanish, 1 tablespoon	— finely chopped

Chopped and diced vegetables can be arranged in layers in soup plate or on regular dinner plate. Dot with half the cottage cheese, cover with sliced tomatoes with balance of cottage cheese in center, topped with green pepper ring and radish in center.

SUGGESTED MENUS

The juice of 1 whole lemon in 6 or 8 ounces of hot water immediately upon arising (no sweetening). The general effect produced will be to flush the liver and the kidneys. (If cold water is used it will be more likely to stimulate the peristaltic action of the intestines.)

In 15 to 30 minutes, drink a glass of fresh orange juice.

Fifteen to 30 minutes later:

Breakfast

One or two 8-ounce glasses fresh raw vegetable juice, either carrot juice as a general mental tonic, or raw potassium (carrot, celery, parsley and spinach) as a blood food or to clear the mind of the effects of "the morning after," if this is needed. Straight celery juice is also good for this.

Carrot and spinach is excellent if the elimination is at all sluggish, or carrot, beet and cucumber juice is a good food for the liver, gall bladder and kidneys.

For many people this juice breakfast will be sufficient. Others will want a little more food, in which case try the following:

No. 1

Bananas, 1 or 2 good ripe (no green on either end)　— sliced.
Sweet cream (preferably raw)
Honey, if sweetening desired
Carrot juice, fresh, 8 ounce glass

Note: If a heavier breakfast is desired, nuts (except peanuts), figs, dates, raisins, persimmons or cottage cheese May be added to the above, either separately or combined to suit the taste.

No. 2

Apples* 1 or 2 medium-sized　— grated or shredded
Sweet cream (preferably raw)
Date sugar or honey for sweetening
Carrot and spinach juice, fresh, 8-ounce glass.

*Many prefer Delicious apples; experiment with different kinds for a few mornings until you find the one best suited to your taste and digestion.

For a more substantial breakfast the above can be covered with 1 or 2 tablespoons of cottage cheese and a few nuts (unsalted almonds, pecans or walnuts).

No. 3

Pears, 1 or 2, grated or shredded, may be used instead of apples in No. 2 breakfast
Carrot, beet and cucumber juice (combined, raw and fresh), 8-ounce glass.

No. 4

Pears, 1 or 2 medium-sized, first layer-grated or diced
Apple, 1 large Delicious, second layer-grated
Date sugar or honey for sweetening, and cream if desired.
Nuts, 1 or 2 tablespoons (any kind except peanuts)
Cottage cheese, I or 2 tablespoons
Carrot and celery juice combined, fresh, 8-oz. glass.

No. 5

Peaches, apricots, berries and other fresh fruits, when in season, either all one kind or
　mixed.
Sweet cream (preferably raw)
Honey for sweetening
Carrot juice, fresh, 8-ounce glass, or carrot and celery or straight celery juice. (These
　are the best juices with this type of breakfast.)

Note: The addition of some figs and dates, whole or chopped, adds variety to any of the above dishes.

No. 6

Sometimes a more substantial breakfast is wanted by one accustomed to a large morning meal that sticks to the ribs. Then we find eggs useful.

Egg yolks, 2 or 4 (no whites) according to size.
Sweet cream, 1 large tablespoon to each 2 yolks.
Vegetable salt

Beat together these ingredients and place in heavy iron skillet which has been previously heated and in which a little butter has been allowed to melt. Cook over a low flame until set and slightly brown underneath, then place skillet under medium high broiler flame until delicately browned on top.

This can be placed on a plate and used as a base to make a variety of dishes, for example: Cover with thin layer of grated apple, or any one of the varieties or combinations of fruit outlined in the preceding breakfast menus, or, place 2 or 3 tablespoonfuls of cottage cheese on the omelet and top this with a layer of grated apple or other fruit.

Carrot juice, fresh, 8-ounce glass, or straight celery juice.
Celery, 2 or 3 stalks, or some lettuce. (This is a good addition to every breakfast.)

Note: Cereals are unnecessary and of no value whatsoever either as nourishment or for energy, unless one is anxious to increase the acid condition of his body.

Prunes, while somewhat acid-forming, have a laxative effect which makes them a popular dish for breakfast. It is not necessary to cook prunes. It is best to soak them for several hours or overnight in tepid water.

Lunch

The best lunch to eat in the middle of the day, to avoid the fatigue which results from the indiscriminate eating of incompatible foods usually served in restaurants, etc., is the following:

No. 1

Vegetable juice, fresh and raw, 1 or 2 pints
Apples, 1 or 2 large, or pears, or bananas, ripe, or 1 or 2 lbs. of grapes, or any other fresh fruit in season in like quantity. One, two or more different fruits may be eaten during lunch.

No. 2

A more substantial lunch:

Cheese*, Swiss, 2 to 4 ounces
Apples, 1 or 2 large juicy
Vegetable juice, fresh and raw, 1 or 2 pints
Celery, several stalks, some spinach, lettuce, watercress or other green vegetable, raw.

*The American Swiss cheese (with holes in it), Wisconsin or similar good quality cheese cut from the large round block, is as good as the imported. (The processed, in squares in packages, is somewhat more acid-forming.)

One week's trial of lunches chosen from these suggestions should prove to the most skeptical that sandwiches, doughnuts and the like are the cause of that let-down condition, that fatigue, which overtakes us in mid-afternoon.

No. 3

Dates, raisins, figs and nuts, handful, separately or mixed.
Celery, 3 or 4 stalks, or some lettuce, spinach, parsley or other green vegetables.
Vegetable juice, fresh raw, 1 pint (straight celery, potassium or carrot)

Note: When a heavier meal is required in the middle of the day, then choose a suggestion from the dinner menus and use the lunch menu in the evening.

It is a good plan, whenever possible, to drink a pint or two of fresh vegetable juices between meals. One pint at least of fresh raw carrot juice in mid-afternoon, for example, works wonders, while in hot weather a pint of straight celery juice helps to keep the body temperature normal and so makes the heat more bearable. The use of ordinary salt in drinking water in hot weather or at any other time has the tendency eventually to harden the arteries.

Dinner

It is an excellent plan to start dinner with at least an 8-ounce glass of fresh raw vegetable juices. They are much more digestible than soup. Straight celery or carrot juice is one of the best juices to drink just before eating a meal.

For the next course, use any one of the salads outlined in the salad section, particularly one of the more elaborate. A sufficient number of salads is given to permit an untiring variety. It is seldom that more food is wanted after eating one of these. However, if dessert is desired, fruit is best. Use any kind that seems most suitable with the salad served.

Remember, think of the saving of labor in dishwashing!

SALAD DRESSINGS

Health Mayonnaise

2 egg yolks
¼ teaspoon vegetable salt
1 teaspoon honey

1 teaspoon lemon juice
1 pint vegetable oil

Mix all ingredients, except oil, in bowl and beat together. Slowly add the oil a drop or two at a time until the mixture is the right consistency. If used on fruit salad a little sweet cream can be beaten in right before using. If used on vegetable salad, the flavor is sometimes improved by the addition of a little sour cream.

Avocado Dressing
Mash a very ripe avocado with fork and add a little Health Mayonnaise, or a few drops of vegetable juice, and beat until smooth and fluffy. If more seasoning is needed add a little vegetable salt and finely grated onion if the dressing is to be used for vegetable salad. If used for fruit salad, add a little honey. (Pepper and other spicy ingredients I also omit entirely as I do not wish to have any irritation of the kidneys or bladder, nor do I want to be troubled with high blood pressure.)

Swiss Cheese Dressing
Grate Swiss cheese and add tomato juice, a few drops at a time, and thoroughly mix into cheese before adding more. Continue this until you have a dressing the consistency of thick whipped cream. This is delicious on any vegetable salad and particularly on tomatoes. It is very rich and should be used in small quantities.

Sour Cream Dressing
1 cup of sour cream, 1 teaspoon of honey and a few drops of lemon juice whipped together until thick.

French Dressing
Olive oil (preferably cold pressed) about ½ pint, ¼ teaspoon powdered kelp or sea lettuce, ¼ teaspoon powdered alfalfa and a little lemon juice and honey. Thoroughly beat together until emulsified and if salt is needed add a little vegetable salt of a good quality.

HOLIDAY DINNERS
Vegetarian-cooked holiday menus for those who feel they must have cooked food at this time. The food combinations are compatible.

Thanksgiving Menu
Appetizer-Small glass fresh apple and celery juice
Celery Hearts Green Ripe Olives Radish Rows

Vegetarian Nut Loaf
Carrot Juice   Carrot and Celery Juice
Fresh buttered green peas   Diced buttered Beets
Cranberry Jelly   Green Salad
Fruit Delight with Whipped Cream

Vegetarian Nut Loaf

9 cups carrot pulp, grated (very fine)
1 cup fresh green Lima Beans (these can be purchased frozen)
2 large onions, finely chapped
10 egg yolks
2 tablespoons finely chopped parsley
1 cup broken Cashew nuts
1 cup finely flaked almonds
6 tablespoons melted butter
3 teaspoons vegetable salt
2½ teaspoons sage
2 teaspoons thyme

Mix grated carrots and other vegetables together in large bowl. Squeeze some of the juice from the grated carrots into the egg yolks, add salt and spices and beat thoroughly and then mix with the vegetables. Add nuts and melted butter and mix very thoroughly. Bake in greased Pyrex loaf pan in moderate oven until done, about 1 hour. Serve on plates in slices just thick enough to hold together. This amount serves 12 people.

Note: Cook the peas and beets until they are barely tender with as little water as possible. Season with little vegetable salt and butter and serve immediately. Do not start to cook them until everything is nearly ready to serve and watch them carefully to make sure that they do not overcooks in which case they will retain their bright color and flavor.

Cranberry Jelly Made With Honey

4 cups washed cranberries (be sure to remove all soft ones or those with spots)
2 cups water
½ cup honey to each cup strained pulp
⅛ cup lemon juice to each 4 cups strained pulp

Cook until berries pop open and are tender. Rub through sieve or collander. Measure sieved pulp and add honey and lemon juice. Cook until it reaches the boiling point and boil hard for 7 minutes, stirring constantly. Remove from fire, pour into sterilized glasses and preserve in the usual way for jelly and jams.

Green Salad

Mix together equal parts of chopped cabbage, spinach, celery, cucumber, green pepper and tomatoes. Sprinkle with olive oil and serve on crisp leaves of lettuce. Garnish with sprigs of parsley.

Fruit Delight

Finely diced pears, dates and chopped walnuts. Sweeten with honey and serve cold topped with whipped cream (also sweetened with honey).

Christmas Dinner

Appetizer-Tomato juice served cold in small cups, to which has been added a bit of very finely grated onion and finely chopped green pepper and celery

Carrot Strips   Ripe Olives   Radishes

Carrot Soufflé

Apple Juice   Carrot and Celery Juice

Steamed Onions   Broccoli

Fresh Green Peas   Stuffed Celery Salad

Cinnamon Apple with Whipped Cream

Carrot Soufflé

6 egg yolks
6 tablespoons water
1/2 teaspoon vegetable salt
2 cups triturated (or finely grated) raw carrot pulp

Thoroughly beat the egg yolks, water and salt and fold in the carrot pulp with a fork. Pour in a greased Pyrex baking dish, square or oblong, about 1½ or 2 inches deep, and bake in a hot oven 450° until done. When a silver knife dipped in cold water and inserted in the soufflé comes out clean it is done. Serve on plates in squares covered with steamed onions. Serves 8 people.

Steamed Onions

The onions can be steamed in their own juice and a bit of olive oil in a casserole dish in the oven while the soufflé is baking. Remove from oven just as soon as tender and sprinkle with yellow grated cheese and a little paprika and place under the broiler just long enough to melt the cheese. Allow 2 medium sized onions for each serving desired. They should be finely chopped before cooking.

Peas and Broccoli

Cook the peas and broccoli just long enough to break up the fibers, remove from fire, season with vegetable salt and butter and serve at once.

Stuffed Celery Salad

Clean and de-string celery. Mix honey with cottage cheese and stuff the celery sticks with mixture. Top with finely grated carrot and finely chopped parsley. Cut crosswise into 2 inch strips and arrange 4 or 5 on crisp lettuce leaves.

Cinnamon Apple with Whipped Cream

Finely grate sweet apples (Delicious are preferable) and season with honey and cinnamon. Serve in sherbet glasses topped with whipped cream sweetened with honey and finely chopped almonds.

No. 1

Salad No. 2.
Carrot juice, fresh raw, 8-ounce glass

Fruit for dessert, for example: 2 or 3 sections of ripe peeled persimmon, ½ pear diced. Top with 1 or 2 teaspoons of whipped cream sweetened with honey, or serve plain with some grated almonds on top.

No. 2

Salad No. 3.
Celery juice straight, fresh raw, 8-ounce glass
Strawberries with honey and cream for dessert.

No. 3

Salad No. 11
Carrot and celery juice, fresh raw, 8-ounce glass.
Peaches, fresh juicy, sprinkled with date sugar or honey.

No. 4

Salad No. 15
Serve with Swiss cheese, 2 or 3 ounces to each serving.
Potassium Broth, fresh raw, 8-ounce glass.
Raspberries, red fresh, served plain or with honey and cream.

No. 5

Salad No. 18
Carrots and Celery juice, fresh raw, 8-ounce glass.
Cherries, sweet ripe, served on stems or pitted and halved in sherbet dishes.

No. 6

Salad No. 21
Carrot, celery and parsley juice, fresh raw, 8-oz. glass.
Grapes (if desired), large purple Tokay, 1 medium sized bunch.

No. 7

Salad No. 27
Serve with Swiss cheese, 2 or 3 ounces to each serving, stuffed olives and celery
 hearts.
Apple and Pomegranate juice, fresh raw, 1 8-oz. glass.
Fresh pineapple strips sprinkled with honey and topped with whipped cream sweetened
 with honey, and grated or finely chopped almonds.

Note: This is a good "Guest" dinner as it is slightly more elaborate than some of the others.

Raw food dinners can always be dressed up and made very colorful and attractive by the addition of radishes, green onions, ripe or stuffed green olives, celery hearts, sliced cucumbers, sliced raw carrots or strips of raw carrot cut thin, lengthwise, sliced raw potatoes, Jerusalem artichokes, whole or sliced, green pepper rings, raw cauliflower hearts, nuts and dates, attractively arranged in odd dishes.

A diet of all raw foods without an abundance of raw vegetable juices, is not sufficient, due to the inability of the body to handle the large volume of raw fiber in vegetables to obtain the necessary amount of the mineral elements.

Therefore, raw foods are just as essential when drinking juices, as raw vegetable juices are when eating raw foods.

If difficulty is experienced in the body handling too much raw food in the beginning, then drink a correspondingly greater quantity of raw vegetable juices and eat plenty of raw fruits, as their fiber is more readily digested and is nearly as efficient.

We must remember that the body will need less food if it is raw than if it is cooked. The calorie method of arranging a meal by calorie portions is nonsense. Raw foods contain only the calories and elements the body requires, particularly if supplemented with plenty of raw vegetable juices.

Overeating

To fill a stomach with more than it is intended to hold for digestive purposes, means stuffing it unduly. Overloading the stomach overtakes all the functions of the body and shortens life.

Did you know that the normal capacity of the average stomach is equivalent to about one quart? Overeating the right kind of foods, even in correct combinations, overworks all the organs of the body. Eat only enough food to be comfortable. Don't think that a stuffed stomach is well-fed. Better far a mite of hunger after a meal than indigestion.

FRESH FRUIT AND RAW VEGETABLE DRINKS
One Pint = 16 Ounces

#1	Carrot	16 oz.	#20	Apple	16 oz.	#32	Carrot	7 oz.
#2	Carrot	7 oz.	#21	Coconut	16 oz.		Beet	3 oz.
	Celery	4 oz.					Lettuce	4 oz.
	Parsley	2 oz.	#22	Grapefruit	16 oz.		Turnip	2 oz.
	Spinach	3 oz.	#23	Lemon	16 oz.	#33	Carrot	10 oz.
#3	Beet & Tops	16 oz.	#24	Orange	16 oz.		Beet	3 oz.
#4	Brussel Sprouts	16 oz.	#25	Pomegranate	16 oz.		Spinach	3 oz.
#5	Cabbage	16 oz.	#26	Carrot	13 oz.	#34	Carrot	11 oz.
#6	Celery	16 oz.		Beet	3 oz.		Cabbage	5 oz.
#7	Cucumber	16 oz.		Note: Use beet tops and roots.		#35	Carrot	7 oz.
#8	Dandelion	16 oz.					Cabbage	4 oz.
#9	Endive (Chicory)	16 oz.	#27	Carrot	7 oz.		Celery	5 oz.
#10	Green Peppers	16 oz.		Apple	6 oz.	#36	Carrot	8oz.
#11	Juice 1 whole Lemon to 1/4 pt. (4 oz.) Horse Radish ground but not pressed.			Beet	3 oz.		Cabbage	4 oz.
			#28	Carrot	8 oz.		Lettuce	4 oz.
				Beet	3 oz.	#37	Carrot	9 oz.
				Celery	5 oz.		Celery	7 oz.
#12	Lettuce	16 oz.	#29	Carrot	11 oz.		Note: If celery tops (greens) are used, then change the proportion to 10 oz. Carrot, 6 oz. Celery.		
#13	Parsley	16 oz.		Beet	3 oz.			
#14	Radish & Tops	16 oz.		Coconut	2 oz.			
#15	Spinach	16 oz.	#30	Carrot	10 oz.			
#16	String Beans	16 oz.		Beet	3 oz.	#38	Carrot	9 oz.
#17	Turnip & Tops	16 oz.		Cucumber	3 oz.		Celery	5 oz.
#18	Watercress	16 oz.	#31	Carrot	9 oz.		Endive (Escarole)	2 oz.
#19	Alfalfa	16 oz.		Beet	3 oz.	#39	Carrot	7 oz.
				Lettuce	4 oz.		Celery	5 oz.
							Lettuce	4 oz.

#40	Carrot	9 oz.	#56	Carrot	9 oz.	#73	Carrot	9 oz.
	Celery	5 oz.		Lettuce	4 oz.		Beet	3 oz.
	Parsley	2 oz.		String Beans	3 oz.		Pomegranate	4 oz.
#41	Carrot	8 oz.	#57	Carrot	6 oz.	#74	Carrot	7 oz.
	Celery	5 oz.		Lettuce	4 oz.		Lettuce	5 oz.
	Radish	3 oz.		String Beans	3 oz.		Pomegranate	4 oz.
#42	Carrot	7 oz.		Brus. Sprouts	3 oz.	#75	Cabbage	5 oz.
	Celery	5 oz.	#58	Carrot	10 oz.		Celery	11 oz.
	Spinach	4 oz.		Lettuce	4 oz.	#76	Celery	8 oz.
#43	Carrot	8 oz.		Turnip	2 oz.		Cucumber	3 oz.
	Celery	6 oz.	#59	Carrot	12 oz.		Parsley	2 oz.
	Turnip	2 oz.		Parsley	4 oz.		Spinach	3 oz.
#44	Carrot	12 oz.	#60	Carrot	11 oz.	#77	Celery	10 oz.
	Cucumber	4 oz.		Radish	5 oz.		Cucumber	4 oz.
#45	Carrot	12 oz.	#61	Carrot	10 oz.		Turnip	2 oz.
	Dandelion	4 oz.		Spinach	6 oz.	#78	Celery	8 oz.
#46	Carrot	9 oz.	#62	Carrot	8 oz.		Dandelion	4 oz.
	Dandelion	3 oz.		Spinach	4 oz.		Spinach	4 oz.
	Lettuce	4 oz.		Turnip	2 oz.	#79	Celery	11 oz.
#47	Carrot	10 oz.		Watercress	2 oz.		Endive (Escarole)	3 oz.
	Dandelion	3 oz.	#63	Carrot	12 oz.		Parsley	2 oz.
	Spinach	3 oz.		Turnip	4 oz.	#80	Celery	7 oz.
#48	Carrot	11 oz.	#64	Carrot	10 oz.		Lettuce	5 oz.
	Dandelion	3 oz.		Turnip	3 oz.		Spinach	4 oz.
	Turnip	2 oz.		Watercress	3 oz.	#81	Celery	10 oz.
#49	Carrot	13 oz.	#65	Carrot	12 oz.		Spinach	4 oz.
	Endive (Escarole)	3 oz.		Watercress	4 oz.		Parsley	2 oz.
#50	Carrot	7 oz.	#66	Carrot	12 oz.	#82	Celery	12 oz.
	Celery	5 oz.		Alfalfa	4 oz.		String Beans	4 oz.
	Endive (Escarole)	2 oz.	#67	Carrot	9 oz.	#83	Brus. Sprouts	7 oz.
	Parsley	2 oz.		Apple	7 oz.		String Beans	9 oz.
#51	Carrot	12 oz.	#68	Carrot	9 oz.	#84	Carrot	6 oz.
	Green Peppers	4 oz.		Fennel	7 oz.		Brus. Sprouts	5 oz.
#52	Carrot	10 oz.	#69	Carrot	13 oz.		String Beans	5 oz.
	Lettuce	6 oz.		Coconut	3 oz.	#85	Carrot	8 oz.
#53	Carrot	9 oz.	#70	Grapefruit	6 oz.		Radish	4 oz.
	Lettuce	4 oz.		Lemon	3 oz.		Lettuce	4 oz.
	Alfalfa	3 oz.		Orange	7 oz.	#86	Carrot	8 oz.
#54	Carrot	7 oz.	#71	Carrot	11 oz.		Radish	4 oz.
	Lettuce	5 oz.		Orange	5 oz.		Watercress	4 oz.
	Cucumber	4 oz.	#72	Carrot	11 oz.	#87	Carrot	6 oz.
#55	Carrot	8 oz.		Pomegranate	5 oz.		Parsnip	4 oz.
	Lettuce	5 oz.					Potato	4 oz.
	Spinach	3 oz.					Watercress	2 oz.

Note: Use Tops and Roots of Beets, Dandelions, Radish and Turnips.

When preparing Carrots cut off the tops ½ inch below the ring where the green stems start and snip off the tail of the carrot.

To remove sprays, etc., we wash vegetables thoroughly with plenty of cold, running water, using a stiff brush when necessary. We prefer to thinly peel all root vegetables unless they are freshly pulled from our own garden and used immediately. When the peeling is removed it improves the flavor and color of the juice.

117

VEGETABLE VALUE CHART

	COMPOUNDS				*VITAMINS*				
	GRAMS				INTER. UNITS	MILLIGRAMS			
Figures based on one pound per category	Distilled Water	Protein	Carbo-hydrates	Fats	Vitamin A	Vitamin C	Thiamin	Riboflavin	Niacin
Alfalfa	393	14	45	.03	199760	799	22.70	187	.49
Artichokes	363	10	77	.51	200	35	1.10	.32	7.10
Asparagus	426	6.40	12.70	.50	2290	84	.46	.51	3.90
Beans-Kidney	380	17.75	38	1	100	0	2.50	.90	10.15
Beans-Lima	310	35	100	3	1500	200	1.18	.60	6.85
Beans-String	400	16	32	.90	3000	100	.38	.50	2.40
Beets	399.30	7.20	64.50	1.12	200	62	.18	.37	2.30
Broccoli	405	16.35	26.80	1.35	16000	600	.51	1.03	.50
Brussels Sprouts	388.50	27.50	36	1.40	3000	525	.63	.97	5
Cabbage	117	8.65	29	.92	1000	250	.31	.33	1.68
Cabbage-Savoy	417	12	25	1.75	1000	200	.30	.30	3.15
Carrots	395	5	44	.92	60000	70	.36	.29	3.15
Cauliflower	414	12.30	21	1.36	410	400	.50	.50	3.30
Celery	429	4.90	16.80	.45	1600	62	.18	.19	1.65
Chard	417	10	19.20	1.30	27120	132	.25	.72	2.20
Chives	409	12	30	2	28000	300	.42	.60	3.60
Corn	342	15	90	5	2500	95	.80	.65	8.50
Cucumbers	435	5.40	13	.45	1400	68	.17	.25	1.12
Dandelion Greens	389	12.75	40	3.15	70000	190	1.10	1.45	.25
Eggplant	423	5.45	23	1.35	100	75	.26	.26	3.10
Garlic	295	30.85	128	.90	20	100	1.30	.45	2.35
Horseradish	348	14.50	78	1.50	0	500	.38	.02	.05
Kale	410	8.60	30	.45	45000	1100	1.15	1.45	12.25
Kohlrabi	408	20	26	.80	200	350	.25	.21	1.65
Leeks	400	11.30	38	1.36	300	100	.60	.50	3
Lettuce	432	6.30	11.20	1.25	5000	76	.38	.36	1.72
Lettuce-Romaine	426	7	19	1.80	10000	115	.38	.52	2.30
Mustard Green	423	9.50	17.80	1.60	22220	308	.34	.70	2.70
Okra	410	10	32	1.30	3000	200	.96	1.12	5.30
Onions	404	7.20	42	1.20	300	89	.18	.23	1.25
Parsley	387	16.70	37	3	40000	550	.60	1.20	5.50
Parsnips	378	7.80	64	3.50	200	95	.45	.53	1.20
Peas	378	18	50	7	3850	165	1.62	.78	.05
Bell Peppers	422	5.40	22	.60	500	600	.38	.38	2.30
Potatoes-White	359	9.50	84	.60	15	132	.63	.26	8.15
Potatoes-Sweet	321	8	122	2.20	39000	200	.62	.43	3.96
Radish	426	5.40	22	.45	75	176	.21	.20	1.65
Spinach	408	15	20	10.50	48000	280	.68	1.15	3.26
Turnips	414	15	65	.50	40	200	.29	.42	2.95
Watercress	423	9.60	12.90	1.20	29000	471	.51	1.09	4.60

MINERALS

GRAMS

Figures based on one pound per category	Calcium	Magnesium	Potassium	Phosphorus	Sulphur	Iron	Silicon	Chlorine	Sodium	Oxygen	Hydrogen	Nitrogen
Alfalfa	7.945	1.497	9.08	1.135	1.316	1.589	.0007	1.271	.681	131	262	2.50
Artichokes	.14	.12	1.95	.57	.20	.16	.01	.16	.44	121	242	1.60
Asparagus	.056	.051	.706	.157	.053	.0025	.008	.004	.005	142	286	1
Beans-Kidney	.21	.12	1.70	.41	.52	.01	.01	.09	.13	126.66	252.34	3
Beans-Lima	.20	.50	4.75	.92	.43	.02	.02	.07	.66	103.34	206.66	6
Beans-String	.54	.45	2.30	.47	.92	.01	.01	.51	.13	133.34	266.66	1.68
Beets	.32	.18	1.94	.62	.32	.05	.40	.46	.46	133.10	266.20	1.22
Broccoli	.46	.11	1.75	.73	.68	.05	.10	.25	.43	135	270	2.63
Brussels Sprouts	.13	.13	1.70	1.10	1.93	.03	.01	.15	.02	129.50	259	3.60
Cabbage	.80	.18	1.92	1.50	1.12	.03	.04	.36	.44	139	278	1.45
Cabbage-Savoy	.21	.63	2.65	1.45	.81	.17	.47	.78	.99	139	278	2
Carrots	.48	.18	1.56	.54	.27	.04	.10	.20	.91	131	262	.85
Cauliflower	.24	.15	1.75	.80	.50	.04	.15	.14	.23	138	276	2.05
Celery	.64	.22	1.54	.47	.21	.05	.14	.57	2.10	143	286	.90
Chard	.367	.271	2.295	.163	.058	.0134	.0312	.063	.613	139	278	1.80
Chives	.95	.24	1.50	.68	.56	.07	.01	.19	.19	136.34	272.66	2
Corn	.08	.41	1.25	1.29	.58	.01	.08	.16	.50	114	228	2.50
Cucumbers	.15	.08	.80	.40	.14	.03	.16	.13	.20	145	290	1
Dandelion Greens	1.70	.70	3.30	.67	.17	.07	.61	.23	.80	129.40	259.6	2.12
Eggplant	.10	.14	1.30	.32	.15	.03	.02	.22	.10	141	282	.91
Garlic	.43	.55	2.40	1.20	1.40	.02	.10	.25	.40	98.34	196.66	5.15
Horseradish	.66	.23	2.30	.42	2.48	.16	1.02	1.02	.04	116	232	2.40
Kale	.80	.20	2.30	1	2.41	.04	.01	.29	.15	136.60	273.30	1.50
Kohlrabi	.80	.57	1.90	.40	.48	.16	.14	.27	.50	136	272	3.60
Leeks	1.08	.02	2	.75	.34	.30	.44	.30	.35	133.34	266.66	1.90
Lettuce	.70	.30	1.80	.45	.18	.25	.39	.37	.36	144	288	1.05
Lettuce-Romaine	.70	.25	1.50	.65	.23	.08	.18	.25	2.09	142	284	1.15
Mustard Green	.581	.086	1.197	.159	.62	.0095	.01	.016	.102	141	282	1.60
Okra	.75	.15	1.10	.41	.33	.01	.10	.05	.45	137	273	1.66
Onions	.59	.14	1	.40	.15	.12	.45	.08	.09	135	270	1.20
Parsley	1.65	.40	3.50	.75	.90	.03	.17	.19	.40	129	258	2.80
Parsnips	.40	.20	2.70	.82	.63	.02	.76	.84	.08	126	252	1.30
Peas	.17	.30	1.60	1.20	.58	.01	.01	.15	.12	126	252	3
Bell Peppers	.30	.54	2.10	.75	.30	.07	.15	.14	.17	141	282	1
Potatoes-White	.13	.25	2.90	.85	.32	.05	.10	.17	.15	120	239	1.60
Potatoes-Sweet	.73	.36	1.45	1.10	.57	.03	.09	.35	.18	107	214	1.60
Radish	.68	.14	1.45	.50	.30	.12	.04	.40	.96	142	284	.95
Spinach	2.15	1.15	3	1.81	1.25	.11	.82	1.14	6.40	136	272	2.50
Turnips	.65	.21	2.70	.84	.55	.03	.05	.38	.33	138	276	2.50
Watercress	1.25	.31	1.60	.80	1.92	.02	.01	.28	.61	141	282	1.60

FRUIT VALUE CHART

| Figures based on one pound per category | COMPOUNDS | | | | VITAMINS | | | | |
| | GRAMS | | | | INTER. UNITS | MILLIGRAMS | | | |
	Distilled Water	Protein	Carbo-hydrates	Fats	Vitamin A	Vitamin C	Thiamin	Riboflavin	Niacin
Acerolas	441	1.80	21.80	1.40	2500	7258	.11	.29	1.90
Apples	387	1.85	73	2.20	500	43	.16	.13	.60
Apricots	384	6.35	60	.20	15000	68	.18	.25	3.31
Avocado	336	9.55	25	85	1500	100	.50	.95	7.50
Bananas	342	5.85	103	2	1000	60	.23	.29	.30
Blackberries	390	5.75	53.50	2.75	2000	125	.18	.24	2.25
Blueberries	378	2.90	63.80	2.10	420	58	.13	.25	1.90
Boysenberries	381	3.20	41.3	.56	590	29	.06	.45	3.40
Cantaloupe	408	3.60	38	.50	15000	183	.24	.18	3.18
Casaba	414	2.70	14.70	Trace	70	29	.10	.07	1.40
Honey Dew	414	2.30	22	.90	120	69	.13	.09	1.80
Muskmelon	408	3.60	38	.50	15000	183	.24	.18	3.18
Cherimoyas	330	5.75	48.50	2.60	50	60	.48	.56	6.30
Cherries	363	5.68	77.20	1.80	1000	65	.30	.30	2.10
Coconut	219	24	84	127	10	0	.28	.22	2.95
Cranberries	405	4.50	43	2	900	100	.21	.12	.52
Currants-Black	360	6	75	.30	1400	1000	.25	.26	1
Currants-Red	390	2.59	60	.18	900	300	.20	.25	.50
Currants-White	387	4.50	60	.20	900	300	.20	.25	.50
Dates	100	9.75	325	5	500	0	.50	.60	12
Figs	360	6.84	86	1.15	550	10	.35	.30	2.15
Grapefruit	399	2.55	45	.25	600	1325	.25	.18	1.20
Grapes	387	5.90	56	4.50	850	48	.26	.20	1.65
Lemons	408	3.30	24.90	.90	50	161	.13	.06	.40
Limes	408	2.70	36.20	.80	50	141	.10	.08	.70
Olives	363	8	12	60	320	10	.10	.09	.10
Oranges	395	6.84	37	.90	1.50	275	.62	.32	2.18
Papaya	399	2.50	46	.50	10000	300	.30	.27	1.75
Peaches	405	3.20	43	.35	7500	58	.14	.33	6.30
Pears	384	3	64	2	200	28	.12	.25	.76
Persimmons	363	2.70	75.10	1.50	10330	42	.11	.08	.40
Plums	369	3.20	81	.05	1750	45	.23	.22	3
Prunes	366	4	80	.20	7200	20	7.30	.80	7.25
Pomegranate	348	1.30	41.70	.80	Trace	10	.07	.07	.70
Pumpkin	408	3.20	20.60	.30	5080	30	.14	.35	1.80
Raspberries-Blk.	381	6.40	60	6	20	100	.21	.52	4.93
Raspberries-Red	390	5.40	56	2.90	800	152	.19	.53	5
Rhubarb	429	1.20	7.60	.20	200	18	.06	.14	.60
Strawberries	408	3	36.60	2.20	260	257	.12	.29	2.60
Tangerines	396	2.70	38.90	.70	1410	105	.20	.05	.40
Tomatoes	427	4.90	19.50	1	5000	150	.38	.30	4
Watermelon	420	2.30	30	.90	3500	90	.18	.20	1.28

MINERALS

GRAMS

Figures based on one pound per category	Calcium	Magnesium	Potassium	Phosphorus	Sulphur	Iron	Silicon	Chlorine	Sodium	Oxygen	Hydrogen	Nitrogen
Acerolas	.045	.049	1.30	.041	.09	.0023	.03	.028	.014	147	294	.32
Apples	.28	.56	.63	.25	.11	.05	.29	.05	.45	129	258	.31
Apricots	.10	.11	1.65	.33	.08	.02	.24	.02	.33	128	256	1.05
Avocado	.45	.50	2.15	1.45	.80	.14	.05	.11	1.50	112	224	1.60
Bananas	.08	.27	1.80	.32	.13	.01	.09	.33	.63	114	228	1
Blackberries	.17	.12	1.10	.45	.15	.07	.23	.05	.10	130	260	.95
Blueberries	.063	.025	.338	.054	.015	.0042	.0001	.00015	.004	126	252	.45
Boysenberries	.086	.082	.386	.086	.017	.0054	.00025	.0002	.005	127	254	.55
Cantaloupe	.12	.12	1.30	.16	.10	.02	.40	.14	.10	136	272	.60
Casaba	.032	.036	.569	.036	.008	.0009	.0002	.0002	.027	136	272	.46
Honey Dew	.040	.036	.00717	.046	.005	.0011	.0003	.00025	.034	136	272	.40
Muskmelon	.12	.12	1.30	.16	.10	.02	.40	.14	.10	136	272	.60
Cherimoyas	.41	.34	2.45	.53	.23	.02	.04	.37	.25	110	220	.93
Cherries	.25	.18	1.70	.53	.10	.07	.30	.05	.07	121	242	.95
Coconut	.45	.50	2.60	2.10	.46	.12	.40	.94	.45	73	146	4
Cranberries	.56	.05	.50	.09	.80	.02	.01	.02	.01	135	270	.75
Currants-Black	.38	.21	1.10	.60	.20	.16	.09	.03	.34	120	240	1
Currants-Red	.15	.10	1.20	.22	.80	.01	.01	.04	.01	130	260	.43
Currants-White	.03	.09	1.40	.13	.37	.01	.01	.03	.02	129	258	.75
Dates	.42	.43	3.80	.36	.45	.05	.01	1.41	.36	33.34	66.66	1.60
Figs	.20	.22	.72	.43	.18	.04	.16	.07	.43	120	240	1.15
Grapefruit	.13	.07	.75	.19	.06	.02	.01	.03	.02	133	266	.42
Grapes	.28	.13	1.80	.40	.15	.05	.06	.04	.04	129	258	.98
Lemons	.079	.0001	.419	.049	.06	.0018	.02	.01	.006	136	272	.85
Limes	.126	.10	.389	.069	.06	.0023	.02	.01	.008	136	272	.46
Olives	.42	.02	3	.07	.05	.03	.03	.01	.40	121	242	1.60
Oranges	.55	.13	1.15	.30	.13	.03	.02	.03	.06	131.66	263.34	1.15
Papaya	.15	.25	1.15	.47	.15	.02	.02	.12	.20	133	266	.40
Peaches	.26	.08	1.12	.34	.18	.03	.01	.05	.17	135	270	6
Pears	.15	.09	.85	.25	.09	.02	.03	.01	.16	126	252	10
Persimmons	.023	.030	.663	.099	.10	.0011	.0001	.00015	.023	121	242	.47
Plums	.31	.27	1.80	.47	.12	.10	.08	.01	.02	107	213	14
Prunes	.40	.17	1.50	.68	.11	.10	.06	.02	.33	122	244	.65
Pomegranate	.008	.0045	.658	.02	.00002	.0008	.01	.03	.008	116	232	.23
Pumpkin	.067	.038	1.08	.14	2.30	.0025	.075	.60	.003	136	272	.55
Raspberries-Blk.	.15	.15	.95	.30	.70	.05	.08	.18	.05	127	254	1.50
Raspberries-Red	.22	.10	1.10	.29	.75	.05	.12	.20	.13	130	260	.90
Rhubarb	.196	.033	.512	.037	.0047	.0016	.007	.014	.004	143	286	.21
Strawberries	.091	.052	.714	.091	.026	.0044	.098	.013	.004	136	272	.50
Tangerines	.134	.035	.423	.06	.032	.0013	.0032	.0033	.007	132	264	.65
Tomatoes	.30	.37	2.20	.29	.14	.03	.05	.38	.89	142	284	.80
Watermelon	.15	.08	.65	.20	.10	.06	.05	.04	.14	140	280	.40

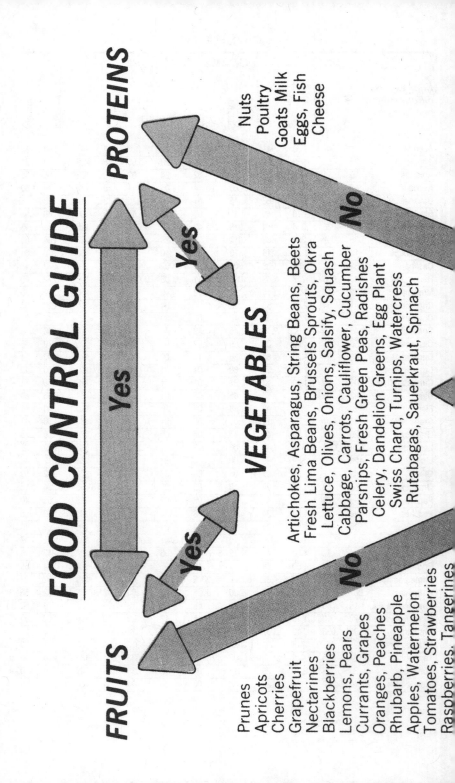

FOOD CONTROL GUIDE

PROTEINS

Nuts
Poultry
Goats Milk
Eggs, Fish
Cheese

No

Yes

Yes

Yes

VEGETABLES

Artichokes, Asparagus, String Beans, Beets
Fresh Lima Beans, Brussels Sprouts, Okra
Lettuce, Olives, Onions, Salsify, Squash
Cabbage, Carrots, Cauliflower, Cucumber
Parsnips, Fresh Green Peas, Radishes
Celery, Dandelion Greens, Egg Plant
Swiss Chard, Turnips, Watercress
Rutabagas, Sauerkraut, Spinach

No

FRUITS

Prunes
Apricots
Cherries
Grapefruit
Nectarines
Blackberries
Lemons, Pears
Currants, Grapes
Oranges, Peaches
Rhubarb, Pineapple
Apples, Watermelon
Tomatoes, Strawberries
Raspberries, Tangerines

CARBOHYDRATES
(SUGAR AND STARCH)

All cold cereals and breakfast foods, popcorn, macaroni, bread, cake, cookies, (flour products), candy, all sugars and syrups.

With meals containing starches and sugars use only these fruits: bananas, dates, figs and raisins.

Note:
Use honey for all sweetening

Use this for your daily guide:

Do not eat any concentrated carbohydrate foods during a meal in which acid or semi-acid fruits or concentrated proteins are included.

No means: Do not combine these foods during the same meal.
Yes means: These foods may be eaten together.

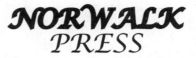

NORWALK
PRESS

Year after year Modern Medical Science continues to prove Dr. Walker is right.

QTY.	TITLE	PRICE	TOTAL
	Diet and Salad	$9.95	
	Fresh Vegetables and Fruit Juices	$9.95	
	Vibrant Health	$9.95	
	Water Can Undermine Your Health	$9.95	
	Become Younger	$9.95	
	Colon Health	$9.95	
	Natural Weight Control	$9.95	
	Foot Relaxation Chart	$6.95	
	Colon Therapy Chart	$6.95	
	Endocrine Glands Chart	$6.95	
		Sub-Total	$
	___ items x $3.95 Each Item (S&H)		$
		TOTAL AMOUNT	$

NAME _____

STREET ADDRESS _____

CITY _____

STATE _____ ZIP _____

To order using this page please xerox the page, make your selection(s), and then calculate your total. Please send your xerox of this page and a check or money order to:

Mail Order Catalog • P.O. Box 180 • Summertown, TN 38483
1-800-695-2241

You may also purchase these health titles from your local bookstore or natural food store.

To find your favorite vegetarian and soyfood products online, visit: www.healthy-eating.com